GREEN AND LEAN COOKBOOK

500 RECIPES

JOHN LARSEN

© Copyright 2021 - All rights reserved.

TABLE OF CONTENTS

Introduction

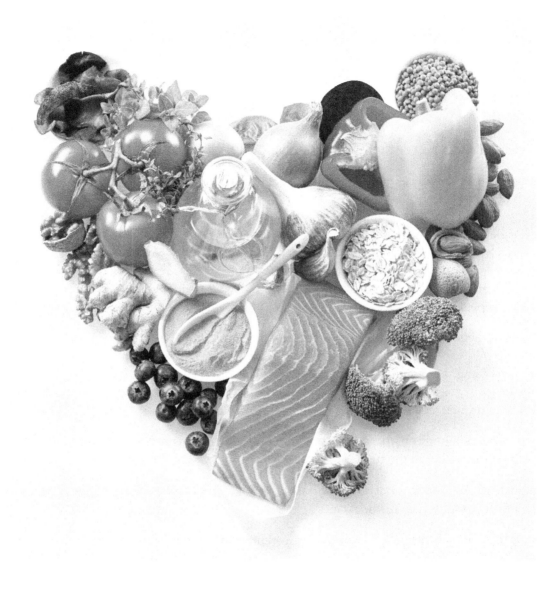

My story begins seven years ago at almost 60 lbs. I was on a mission to transform my body into something healthier. I was introduced to many new diets and exercise programs, some of which failed to achieve any significant results, and others made a small contribution to my weight loss. The internet is full of amazing diets that promise to help me lose a lot of weight with little effort, but fail to deliver. Nothing came close to achieving my weight loss goal. Then I discovered the Lean and Green diet. I was thrilled with the supplies I received for the plan I chose, but the Lean and Green meals are proving to be a tough nut to crack because I don't know what to prepare that meets the diet's recommendations.

I wish I could take the guesswork out of the whole process to focus on taking the portions of food provided and not spend too much time following the nutritional information. However, with the guidance of my dietitian, I was able to combine some vegetable recipes to make a healthy diet. Despite this, the process was nerve-wracking. I documented the recipes and diets, followed the diet strictly and experienced excellent results. I lost weight beyond my expectations and developed a new relationship with food. Six years later, I am still active, strong and maintaining a healthy weight. Eating Lean & Green has become part of my lifestyle, and I have documented my Lean and Green diet in this cookbook to help you make a healthy choice with your diet .

I have struggled with an unhealthy body weight for most of my life, the inspiration to write this diet book comes from a deep desire to help others on a similar journey. I'm excited to share nutritious and healthy Lean and Green diets that are also incredibly satisfying and delicious.As you know, the Lean and Green diet is a commercial diet, but it is considered one of the most popular diets that have brought many benefits over the three decades. Lean and Green is a home cooked meal option that encourages weight loss through strict homemade green recipes to improve blood lipids, sugar levels and better overall health. Lean and Green is an easy, affordable, and long-lasting diet to lose weight quickly and effectively. This book will be your guide so that you can enjoy delicious and healthy food that can improve your health.

Are you tired of diets that promise results but take a huge amount of time and effort to plan? Or are you looking for a diet that will help you lose unnecessary weight in a fast, safe and convenient way? You can finally stop agonizing over losing time, money or inspiration with this Lean and Green cookbook. The recipes in this book will help you lose weight in the shortest possible time, and will also boost your confidence and promote motivation to continue.

The recipes contain ingredients that will help you lose weight and maintain good overall health without worrying about regaining the weight in the future.

This book helps you develop a healthy relationship with food while educating you with the health benefits and nutritional information in each of the recipes.

Soon, preparing a healthy diet will be a breeze, as you now have the information on how to prepare meals that fit your needs.

And now, with this handy Lean and Green book, your days of confusion about what to prepare are over, because this comprehensive cookbook is prepared to help you meet all your Lean and Green needs.

Losing weight doesn't have to taste bad or look bad. This book will help you understand Lean and Green so that you can enjoy delicious healthy foods that can improve your health and learn new recipes to make your meals more exciting. This book guides you with detailed information and a mixture of different recipes that will help you in your quest for a healthier life.

This book is ideal for people who don't have time for very complex preparations and are looking for quick, healthy recipes that make little time in the kitchen. These recipes are full of nutrients and ingredients such as lean proteins, vegetables, healthy fats, non-starchy vegetables and spices, ideal for those who want a delicious low-fat diet that is quick and easy to prepare. You no longer have to live on unhealthy fast food; this cookbook offers tasty home cooking recipes that are perfect for you.

One of the vital components to losing weight is eating diets that are delicious and nutrient-dense. The Lean and Green Cookbook offers a wide range of healthy choices to satisfy your cravings, allowing you to stick to healthy diets while remaining completely satisfied. The Lean and Green Cookbook is a simple collection of diets to which you can add fresh vegetables. With these simple recipes, you won't have to break the bank in order to eat healthy.

Food varieties allowed in your Lean and Green meal include:

Meat: Turkey, chicken, lean beef, game, pork chop or tenderloin, lamb, ground beef (at least 85% lean).

Fish and Shellfish: Salmon, tuna, halibut, trout, scallops, lobster, crab, shrimp.

Eggs: Whole eggs, eggshells, egg whites.

Soy products: Tofu.

Vegetable oils: Olive oil, canola, flaxseed, walnuts.

Low-carb vegetables: Spinach, chard greens, mushrooms, eggplant, celery, cucumbers, cabbage, broccoli, cauliflower, zucchini, peppers, spaghetti.

Sugar free snacks: popsicles, mints, jelly, chewing gum

Sugar-free drinks: unsweetened almond milk, coffee, tea, water.

Other healthy fats: Almonds, low carb salad dressings, avocados, low fat margarine, pistachios.

Food varieties to avoid in your Lean and Green meal include:

Fried foods: fried foods, sweets such as pastries

Refined grains: Biscuits, white bread, pancakes, flour tortillas, pasta crackers, white rice, cookies, cakes.

Fats: Coconut oil, butter

Alcohol: All varieties

Whole Dairy Products: Milk, cheese, yogurt

Sugary drinks: Soda juices, energy drinks, sports drinks.

Chapter 1:

Weekly Shopping List

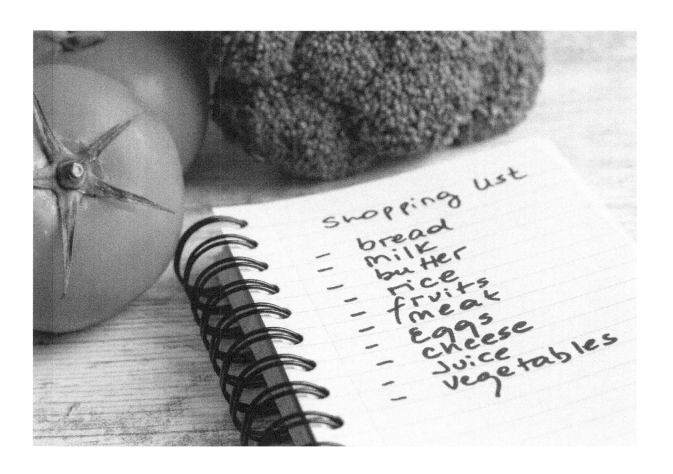

Vegetables:

- Lettuce
- Spinach
- Celery
- Arugula
- Cabbage
- Eggplant
- Cauliflower
- Kale
- Asparagus
- Turnips
- Broccoli
- Mushrooms

Fish:

- Cod
- Tuna
- Mahi-mahi
- Salmon

Shellfish:

- Crab
- Shrimp
- Scallop

Poultry:

- Chicken
- Chicken Breast

Meat:

- Pork Chop/Tenderloin
- Lamb
- Lean beef

Meatleass Options:

- Eggs
- Tofu

Herbs/Spices:

- Basil
- Parsley
- unsweetened almond milk

- Pepper
- Rosemary
- Spice mixes
- Nutmeg
- Bay leaf
- Cloves
- Ginger
- Paprika
- Garlic Powder
- Oregano
- Dill seed
- Salt

Sauces/Syrups:

- Oyster sauce
- Tomato Paste
- Worcestershire sauce
- Soy sauce
- Vinegar
- Catsup

Baking/Cooking Ingredients:

- Baking powder
- Baking soda
- Pine nuts
- Sesaame seeds
- Sunflower seeds
- Baker's yeast

Oils:

- Walnut
- Flaxseed
- olive oil
- canola

Sugar-free beverages:

- Coffee
- Tea
- water

Chapter 2:

Breakfast Recipes

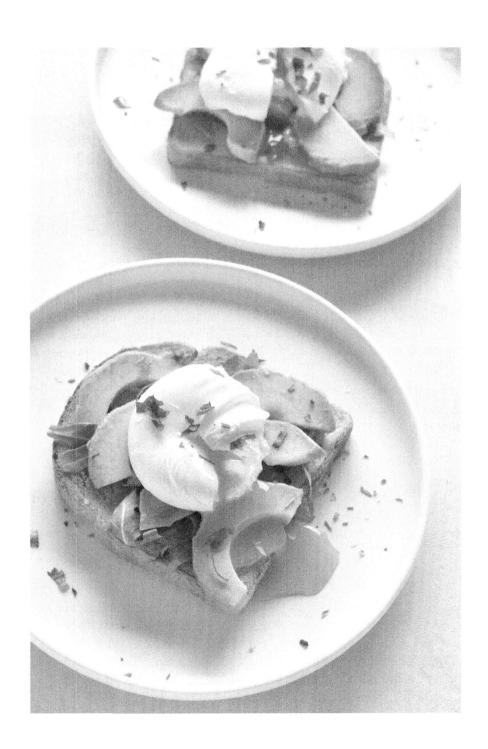

1. Eggs and Avocado Toast

Prep Time: 15 minutes
Cook Time: 4 minutes
Portions: 4
Ingredients:
4 whole-wheat bread slices
4 hard-boiled eggs
1/4 tsp. lemon juice
1 avocado
Salt
ground black pepper
Directions:
Pit the avocado then peel and chop it. To the same with the eggs
In a bowl, add the avocado, and with a fork, mash it. Combine lemon juice, pepper, and salt in a bowl and set aside
Using a nonstick frying pan, on medium-high heat, toast the slices for about 2 minutes per side.
Spread the avocado mixture over each slice evenly.
Top each with egg slices and serve immediately.
Nutrition:
Calories: 162 kcal
Protein: 7.52 g
Fat: 12.69 g
Carbohydrates: 5.93 g

2. Eggless Scramble

Prep Time: 10 minutes
Cook Time: 8 minutes
Portions: 2
Ingredients:
2 3/4 cup baby spinach
1/3 cup vegetable broth
1/4 lb. tofu
2 tsp. low-sodium soy sauce
1 garlic clove
1 tsp. turmeric
1 tbsp. olive oil
1 tsp. lemon juice

Directions:
Mince the garlic. Drain, press, and crumble the tofu. In a frying pan, heat the olive oil over medium-high heat and sauté the garlic for about 1 minute.
Add the tofu and cook for about 2–3 minutes, slowly adding the broth.
Add the spinach, soy sauce, and turmeric, and stir fry for about 3–4 minutes or until all the liquid is absorbed.

Stir in the lemon juice and remove it from the heat. Serve immediately.
Nutrition:
Calories: 265 kcal
Protein: 14.89 g
Fat: 20.58 g
Carbohydrates: 10.12 g

3. Baked Eggs

Prep Time: 10 minutes
Cook Time: 9 minutes
Portions: 6
Ingredients:
3/4 cup low-fat Parmesan cheese
1/2 cup heavy cream
2 cup spinach
12 large eggs
Salt
Pepper
Directions:
Finely chop the spinach and shred the parmesan cheese. Preheat your oven to 425°F.
Grease a 12-cup muffin tin. Divide spinach in each muffin cup. Crack an egg over spinach into each cup and drizzle with heavy cream.
Sprinkle with salt, pepper, and parmesan cheese.
Bake for approximately 7-9 minutes or until the desired doneness of eggs. Serve right away.
Nutrition:
Calories: 201 kcal
Protein: 10.69 g
Fat: 16.34 g
Carbohydrates: 2.69 g

4. Banana and Pumpkin Waffles

Prep Time: 15 minutes
Cook Time: 5 minutes
Portions: 4
Ingredients:
2 medium bananas
11/2 tsp. ground cinnamon
1/2 cup coconut flour
2 tbsp. olive oil
1/2 tsp. ground cloves
3/4 tsp. ground ginger
1 tsp. baking soda
1/2 tsp. ground nutmeg
1/2 cup almond flour
5 large eggs
3/4 cup almond milk
1/2 cup pumpkin puree

Salt

Directions:
Peel and slice the bananas.
Preheat the waffle iron, and after that, grease it.
In a sizable bowl, mix flour, baking soda, and spices.
In a blender, put the remaining ingredients and pulse till smooth.
Add flour mixture and pulse till smooth.
In preheated waffle iron, add the required quantity of mixture.
Cook approximately 4-5 minutes.
Repeat using the remaining mixture.
Nutrition:
Calories: 357.2 kcal Protein: 14 g
Fat: 28.5 g Carbohydrates: 19.7 g

5. Cashew and Blueberry Waffles
Prep Time: 15 minutes
Cook Time: 4-5 minutes
Portions: 5
Ingredients:
1/2 cup unsweetened almond milk
3 tbsp. coconut flour
3 tbsp. honey
1 cup blueberries
Salt
3 organic eggs
1/4 cup coconut oil
1/2 tsp. vanilla flavor
1 cup raw cashews
1 tsp. baking soda
Directions:
Melt the coconut oil.
Preheat the waffle iron and then grease it.
In a mixer, add cashews and pulse till flour-like consistency forms.
Transfer the cashew flour to a big bowl.
Add almond flour, baking soda, and salt and mix well.
In another bowl, put the remaining ingredients and beat till well combined.
Put the egg mixture into the flour mixture, then mix till well combined.
Fold in blueberries.
In preheated waffle iron, add the required amount of mixture.
Cook for around 4-5 minutes.
Repeat with the remaining mixture.
Nutrition:
Calories: 432 kcal

Protein: 13 g Fat: 32 g
Carbohydrates: 32 g

6. Cheddar and Chive Soufflés
Prep Time: 10 minutes
Cook Time: 25 minutes
Portions: 8
Ingredients:
1/2 cup almond flour
1/4 cup chives
1 tsp. salt
1/2 tsp. xanthan gum
1 tsp. ground mustard
1/4 tsp. cayenne pepper
1/2 tsp. cracked black pepper
3/4 cup heavy cream
2 cup cheddar cheese
1/2 cup baking powder
6 organic eggs
Directions:
Chop the chives.
Shred the cheddar cheese.
Switch on the oven, then set its temperature to 350°F and let it preheat.
Take a medium bowl, add flour in it, add remaining ingredients, except for baking powder and eggs, and whisk until combined.
Separate egg yolks and egg whites between two bowls, add egg yolks in the flour mixture and whisk until incorporated.
Add baking powder into the egg whites and beat with an electric mixer until stiff peaks form and then stir egg whites into the flour mixture until well mixed.
Divide the batter evenly between eight ramekins and then bake for 25 minutes until done.
Serve straight away or store in the refrigerator until ready to eat.
Nutrition:
Calories: 288 kcal
Protein: 14 g
Fat: 21 g
Carbohydrates: 3 g

7. Broccoli Waffles
Prep Time: 10 minutes
Cook Time: 8 minutes
Portions: 2
Ingredients:
1/3 cup broccoli
1/2 tsp. dried onion
1 egg

1/4 cup low-fat Cheddar cheese
1/2 tsp. garlic powder
Salt
Pepper
Directions:
Finely chop the broccoli.
Shred the cheddar and mince the onions.
Preheat a mini waffle iron and then grease it.
In a medium bowl, place all ingredients and mix until well combined.
Place 1/2 of the mixture into preheated waffle iron and cook for about 3-4 minutes or until golden brown.
Repeat with the remaining mixture.
Serve warm.
Nutrition:
Calories: 156 kcal
Protein: 10.59 g
Fat: 8.53 g
Carbohydrates: 10.59 g

8. Kale Scramble

Prep Time: 10 minutes
Cook Time: 6 minutes
Portions: 2
Ingredients:
1 cup kale
1/8 tsp. ground turmeric
1/8 tsp. red pepper flakes
4 eggs
1 tbsp. water
2 tsp. olive oil
Salt
Black Pepper
Directions:
Crush the pepper flakes.
Remove the ribs and chop the kale.
In a bowl, add the eggs, turmeric, red pepper flakes, salt, pepper, and water and whisk until foamy.
In a skillet, heat the oil over medium heat
Add the egg mixture and stir to combine.
Immediately reduce the heat to medium-low and cook for about 1-2 minutes, stirring frequently.
Stir in the kale and cook for about 3-4 minutes, stirring frequently.
Remove from the heat and serve immediately.
Nutrition:
Calories: 314 kcal
Protein: 18.8 g
Fat: 23.91 g

Carbohydrates: 5.27 g

9. Cheesy Spinach Waffles

Prep Time: 10 minutes
Cook Time: 20 minutes
Portions: 4
Ingredients:
4 oz. frozen spinach
1/2 cup part-skim Mozzarella cheese
1 large egg
1 cup ricotta cheese
1/4 cup low-fat grated Parmesan cheese
1 garlic clove
Salt
Pepper
Directions:
Crumble the ricotta cheese. Shred the mozzarella. Mince the garlic Preheat a mini waffle iron and then grease it. In a bowl, add all the ingredients and beat until well combined. Place 1/4 of the mixture into preheated waffle iron and cook for about 4-5 minutes or until golden brown.
Repeat with the remaining mixture.
Serve warm.
Nutrition:
Calories: 178 kcal
Protein: 12.49 g
Fat: 11.82 g
Carbohydrates: 6.14 g

10. Cheesy Flax and Hemp Seeds Muffins

Prep Time: 5 minutes
Cook Time: 30 minutes
Portions: 2
Ingredients:
1/4 cup cottage cheese, low-fat
1/4 cup raw hemp seeds
1/4 cup almond meal
1/8 cup flax seeds meal
1/4 tsp. baking powder
3 eggs
1/8 cup nutritional yeast flakes
1/4 cup parmesan cheese
1/4 cup scallion
Salt
1 tbsp. olive oil
Directions:
Switch on the oven, then set it at 360°F and let it preheat. Meanwhile, take two ramekins, grease them with oil, and set them aside until required.

Take a medium bowl, add flax seeds, hemp seeds, and almond meal, and then stir in salt and baking powder until mixed. Crack eggs in another bowl, add yeast, cottage cheese, and parmesan, stir well until combined, and then stir this mixture into the almond meal mixture until incorporated.

Thinly slice the scallions. Fold the in, and then distribute the mixture between prepared ramekins and bake for 30 minutes until muffins are firm and the top is nicely golden brown.

When done, take out the muffins from the ramekins and let them cool completely on a wire rack.

For meal prepping, wrap each muffin with a paper towel and refrigerate for up to thirty-four days.

When ready to eat, reheat muffins in the microwave until hot and then serve.

Nutrition:
Calories: 179 kcal
Protein: 15.4 g
Fat: 10.9 g
Carbohydrates: 6.9 g

11. Flaxseed Porridge with Cinnamon

Prep Time: 10 minutes
Cook Time: 5 minutes
Portions: 4
Ingredients:
2 tbsp. flaxseed meal
1 tsp. cinnamon
1/2 cup shredded coconut
1 tbsp. unsalted butter
11/2 tsp. stevia
2 tbsp. flaxseed oatmeal
1 cup heavy cream
2 cups of water
Directions:
Take a medium pot, place it over low heat, add all the ingredients in it, stir until mixed and bring the mixture to boil.

When the mixture has boiled, remove the pot from heat, stir it well and divide it evenly between four bowls.

Let porridge rest for 10 minutes until slightly thicken and then serve.

Nutrition:
Calories: 171 kcal
Protein: 2 g
Fat: 16 g
Carbohydrates: 6 g

12. Cinnamon Pancakes with Coconut

Prep Time: 5 minutes
Cook Time: 18 minutes
Portions: 2
Ingredients:
2 eggs
1/4 cup shredded coconut
1 tbsp. almond flour
1/4 cup shredded coconut
1 tsp. cinnamon
1/2 tbsp. erythritol
2 oz. cream cheese
4 tbsp. stevia
1/2 tbsp. olive oil
1/8 tsp. salt
Directions:
Crack eggs in a bowl, beat until fluffy and then beat in flour and cream cheese until smooth.

Add remaining ingredients and then stir until well combined.

Take a frying pan, place it over medium heat, grease it with oil, then pour in half of the batter and cook for 3 to 4 minutes per side until the pancake has cooked and nicely golden brown.

Transfer pancake to a plate and cook another pancake in the same manner by using the remaining batter.

Sprinkle coconut on top of cooked pancakes and serve.

Nutrition:
Calories: 575 kcal
Protein: 19 g
Fat: 51 g
Carbohydrates: 3.5 g

13. Banana Cashew Toast

Prep Time: 10 minutes
Cook Time: 0 minutes
Portions: 3
Ingredients:
2 ripe medium-sized bananas
1 cup roasted cashews
cinnamon
2 tsp. flax meals
4 pieces of oat bread
2 tsp. honey
Salt
Directions:

Peel and slice the bananas.

Toast the bread.

In a food processor, puree the salt and cashews until they are smooth. Use the puree as a spread on the toasts.

On top of the spread, arrange a layer of bananas.

Add flax meals and a dash of cinnamon on top of the bananas.

Top the toast with honey.

Nutrition:

Calories: 634 kcal

Protein: 13.42 g

Fat: 47.6 g

Carbohydrates: 48.02 g

14. Apple Oatmeal

Prep Time: 10 minutes

Cook Time: 5 minutes

Portions: 2

Ingredients:

1 apple

2/3 cup rolled oats

1 cup water

1 cup of any non-fat milk

1 tsp. ground cinnamon

1/4 cup apple juice

Directions:

Peeled or unpeeled, chop the apple.

Place the water, juice, and apple in a deep pot. Bring to a boil over medium heat.

Add the oats and cinnamon. Bring to another boil.

Lower the heat temperature and let it simmer for 3 minutes or until it is thick.

Divide the serving into two and serve with milk.

Nutrition:

Calories: 277 kcal

Protein: 12.69 g

Fat: 7.69 g

Carbohydrates: 52.71 g

15. Strawberry Yogurt treats

Prep Time: 10 minutes

Cook Time: 0 minutes

Portions: 2

Ingredients:

4 cup 0% fat plain Greek yogurt

1 cup strawberries

8 tbsp. of flax meal

4 tbsp. honey

8 tbsp. walnuts

Directions:

Chop the walnuts.

Wash and slice the strawberries.

Distribute 2 cups of the yogurt into your serving bowls.

Neatly layer the flax meal and the walnut in the middle.

Add a drizzle of half of the honey before covering it with the last layer of yogurt.

Add the honey on top of the yogurt to add color when you serve.

Nutrition:

Calories: 733 kcal

Protein: 38.42 g

Fat: 30.57 g

Carbohydrates: 83.44 g

16. Cold Banana Breakfast

Prep Time: 10 minutes

Cook Time: -

Portions: 2

Ingredients:

1/2 cup cold milk

4 tbsp. sesame seeds

2 tbsp. flaxseeds

4 tbsp. sunflower seeds

2 tbsp. ground coconut

1 large banana

Directions:

Mix the milk and honey in your breakfast bowl.

Use your coffee grinder to grind all the seeds.

Add the ground seeds to the honey and milk mixture.

Peel and slice the banana. Place the slices neatly on top.

Sprinkle the ground coconuts for added flavor.

Nutrition:

Calories: 393 kcal

Protein: 14.85 g

Fat: 27.63 g

Carbohydrates: 27.37 g

17. Swiss chard and Spinach with Egg

Prep Time: 5 minutes

Cook Time: 10 minutes

Portions: 4

Ingredients:

20 pieces Swiss chard leaves

4 pieces of rice bread

20 pieces spinach leaves

4 tbsp. parsley
4 egg whites
1 tsp. olive oil
salt
pepper
dried mint

Directions:

Bring to a boil 2 cups of water in a pan just below the boiling point. Open an egg; separate the whites from the yolks. Put the whites in a small bowl. Lower the bowl towards the heated water, and gently pour the egg into the pan.

Do the same with the other eggs. Poach the eggs for 4 minutes.

After that, gently take the eggs one at a time and transfer them to a plate.

Do the same with the remaining 2 eggs.

Chop the parsley and sauté the leaves in a pan for 6 minutes. Toast the bread while doing this.

When done, make a layer of the sautéed greens and the chopped parsley on top of the toasted rice bread. Put the poached eggs above the bed of greens. Sprinkle each serving with ground pepper, sea salt, and dried mint

Nutrition:

Calories: 49 kcal
Protein: 5.31 g
Fat: 2.73 g
Carbohydrates: 0.48 g

18. Lemon Yogurt Sauce Breakfast

Prep Time: 10 minutes
Cook Time: 0 minutes
Portions: 2

Ingredients:

11/2 cup barley
1 cup bean sprouts
1/3 cup cheese
1/4 cup almonds
1/4 tsp. salt
1 small avocado
1/2 tsp. salt
1/4 tsp. black pepper
Lemon Yogurt Sauce
1 cup Greek plain yogurt
1 tsp. lemon zest
1 tsp. lemon juice
1/4 cup fresh mint
salt
pepper

Directions:

First, prepare the Lemon Yogurt Sauce: Combine the plain yogurt, finely grated lemon zest and juice, chopped mint, salt, and pepper in a bowl and stir to blend well. Cover and refrigerate until ready to serve. Cook the barley. Toast the almonds using a baking sheet.

Peel, pit and thinly slice the avocado.

Next, prepare the barley bowl: In a small mixing bowl, combine the cooked barley, bean sprouts, cheese, sliced almonds, and salt. Stir to mix well.

Divide barley mixture into 2 serving bowls. Top each barley bowl with 2 tbsp. lemon yogurt sauce and avocado. Put a pinch of salt and pepper to taste, serve,

Enjoy!

Nutrition:

Calories: 432 kcal
Protein: 13.6 g
Fat: 23.37 g
Carbohydrates: 47.62 g

19. Cherry Almond Parfait

Prep Time: 25 minutes
Cook Time: 5 minutes
Portions: 2

Ingredients:

1 cup red cherries
2 tbsp. almond syrup
2 tbsp. coconut palm sugar
1 tsp. lemon juice
2 cup Greek plain yogurt
2 tbsp. almonds
4 tbsp. granola

Directions:

Place a saucepan over medium-high heat and combine pitted cherries, almond syrup, sugar, lemon juice, and 1 tbsp. of water. Stir to combine, then place it to simmer, constantly stirring until sugar is dissolved. Continue to simmer for further 5 minutes until liquid starts to turn into a syrupy mixture, but the cherries are still holding firm.

Place the mixture in a bowl and let cool for 5 minutes at room temperature, then bring it in the refrigerator to chill until it is completely cold.

Place 1 cup of Greek yogurt into 2 serving bowls and spoon 1/2 of the cherries and their syrupy juices over the yogurt.

Garnish with sliced almonds or granola, if desired.

Serve immediately.
Nutrition:
Calories: 185 kcal
Protein: 4.75 g
Fat: 4.88 g
Carbohydrates: 33.07 g

20. Strawberry-Oat-Chocolate Chip Muffins

Prep Time: 10 minutes
Cook Time: 23 minutes
Portions: 12
Ingredients:
3 large ripe bananas
1/2 cup unsweetened vanilla almond milk
11/4 cup whole wheat pastry flour
1/3 cup mini chocolate chips
1 tbsp. honey
3/4 tsp. baking soda
1/4 tsp. salt
1 tbsp. olive oil
1/2 tsp. baking powder
1 tsp. vanilla
1 egg
1 egg white
1 cup rolled oats
1/3 cup nonfat plain Greek yogurt
2/3 cup strawberries
4 strawberries, sliced for garnish
Directions:
Set the oven to 350°F and lightly grease a standard 12-cup muffin pan or grease with paper liners. In a large-sized mixing bowl, combine flour, oats, baking powder, baking soda, and salt. Stir to blend. Set aside the 2 tbsp. of the mixture. In a separate huge mixing bowl, combine the mashed banana, olive oil, honey, and vanilla. Next, beat in the egg and egg white and beat until combined. Now add in Greek yogurt and almond milk and beat with an electric mixer on low until smooth. Gradually put wet ingredients to dry ingredients and blend until just combined, but don't over mix the batter as it will make the muffins firm. Fill each muffin cup 2/3 full of batter. Gently tap the pan on the counter to even out the batter. Place a thin slice of strawberry onto each muffin, if desired. Put the pan in the oven, and then cook for 18 to 23 minutes, until a toothpick placed in the center of the muffins comes out clean. Take off from the oven and

let sit for 5 to 10 minutes in the pan before placing on a cooling rack.
Nutrition:
Calories: 91 kcal
Protein: 4.02 g
Fat: 2.63 g
Carbohydrates: 16.31 g

21. Blueberry Breakfast Sundae

Prep Time: 10 minutes
Cook Time: 0 minutes
Portions: 2
Ingredients:
2 cup vanilla Greek yogurt
2 cup bran flakes
1/4 cup blueberries
2 tbsp. almonds
2 tbsp. pecans
2 tbsp. cranberries
Directions:
In a bowl, place 1 cup yogurt, and one cup of bran flakes. Top with 1/8 cup fresh blueberries, followed by 1 tbsp. each of sliced almonds, chopped pecans, and dried cranberries. Repeat using the remaining ingredients to make a second serving. Serve immediately.
Nutrition:
Calories: 420 kcal
Protein: 21.12 g
Fat: 13.58 g
Carbohydrates: 59.8 g

22. Cinnamon-Apple Granola with Greek Yogurt

Prep Time: 5 minutes
Cook Time: 10 minutes
Portions: 2
Ingredients:
1 cup Greek plain yogurt
2 tsp. honey
1 tsp. ground cinnamon
1/2 apple
1 tbsp. almond flour
2 tbsp. vanilla protein powder
1/8 cup applesauce
1/2 cup raw walnuts
2 tsp. almond butter
1/16 tsp. vanilla extract
1/2 cup raw almonds
Salt

Directions:

In a bowl, mix well the chopped almonds, chopped walnuts, diced apple, vanilla protein powder, almond flour, cinnamon and salt.

In a second bowl, combine the apple sauce, almond butter, honey, and vanilla extract. Mix well. Pour the bowl with the nuts into the bowl with the wet ingredients and blend thoroughly. Make sure all dry ingredients get coated.

Place the granola mixture onto a parchment paper-lined baking sheet and bake until the desired crunch is obtained for approximately 8 to 10 minutes. Take off from the oven and let cool or eat hot. Place 1/2 cup of each Greek yogurt into two bowls. Divide the granola and sprinkle over the yogurt in each bowl. Serve immediately.

Nutrition:
Calories: 312 kcal
Protein: 11.72 g
Fat: 22.37 g
Carbohydrates: 19.92 g

23. Egg-Tilla

Prep Time: 5 minutes
Cook Time: 5 minutes
Portions: 2

Ingredients:
(2) 8-inch whole wheat tortillas
2 hard-boiled eggs
2 slices of Canadian bacon
1 oz. slice of cheddar cheese
2 tbsp. salsa

Directions:
Prepare the hardboiled eggs.
Put 1 tortilla on a plate, top with a slice of Canadian bacon, the sliced egg, and a slice of cheddar cheese. Roll the tortilla up. Repeat with the remaining ingredients to prepare the second burrito.
Serve immediately with 1 tbsp. Salsa.

Nutrition:
Calories: 741 kcal Protein: 36.12 g
Fat: 30.75 g Carbohydrates: 79.37 g

24. Oatmeal-Applesauce Muffins

Prep Time: 15 minutes
Cook Time: 25 minutes
Portions: 12
Ingredients:

Topping
1/4 cup rolled oats
1 tbsp. brown sugar
1/8 tsp. cinnamon
1 tbsp. unsalted butter
Muffins
1/2 cup brown sugar
2 egg whites
1 cup old fashioned rolled oats
1 cup nonfat milk
1 cup whole wheat flour
1/2 cup unsweetened applesauce
1 tsp. Baking powder
1/2 tsp. Cinnamon
1/2 tsp. sugar
raisins
1/2 tsp. Salt
1/2 tsp. Baking soda

Directions:
Presoak the oats in milk for 1 hour.
Set the oven to 400°F and grease a standard 12-cup muffin pan with Cooking spray or use paper liners.
In a mixing bowl, combine oat-milk mixture, applesauce, and egg whites. Blend well and set aside. In a separate bowl, put together the whole wheat flour, brown sugar, baking powder, baking soda, salt, sugar, and cinnamon and mix.
Gradually put wet ingredients to dry ingredients and blend until just combined, but don't over mix the batter as it will make the muffins firm. Add raisins or nuts (opt.).
Prepare the topping: In a small bowl, whisk together the oats, brown sugar, and cinnamon. Add in melted butter and toss gently with a fork to coat ingredients. Fill each muffin cup 2/3 full of batter. Sprinkle topping on the top of each batter-filled muffin cup. Tap the pan gently on the counter to even out the batter. Place muffin pan in preheated oven and cook for 20 to 25 minutes or until a toothpick put in the middle of one of the muffins comes out clean. Take off from the oven and let sit for 5 minutes before serving.

Nutrition:
Calories: 115 kcal Protein: 5.06 g
Fat: 2.57 g Carbohydrates: 22.33 g

25. Banana Vegan Pancakes

Prep Time: 5 minutes
Cook Time: 5 minutes
Portions: 12

Ingredients:
2 ripe bananas
11/4 cup old fashioned oats
2 tsp. Baking powder
1/2 tsp. salt
1/2 cup organic whole wheat flour
11/2 cup soymilk

Directions:
To begin, heat griddle or skillet over medium heat.
Next, place all ingredients, except for the banana, into a blender and process until smooth. Add the bananas to the blender and blend until smooth.
Lightly grease griddle with olive or coconut oil, then pour 1/4 cup of batter onto griddle and cook for at least 2 to 3 minutes, then flip and cook for about 2 minutes or up to the pancake is golden brown and cooked through.
Repeat the process with the remaining batter.

Nutrition:
Calories: 59 kcal Protein: 3.49 g
Fat: 1.48 g Carbohydrates: 11.52 g

26. Surprise Muffins
Prep Time: 15 minutes
Cook Time: 25 minutes
Portions: 12

Ingredients:
3 ripe bananas
6 tbsp. creamy peanut butter
1/2 tsp. salt
3/4 cup light brown sugar
2 large eggs
1 cup low-fat buttermilk
1 1/2 cup all-purpose flour
1 tsp. Baking powder
1 cup old-fashioned oats
1/2 tsp. Baking soda
2 tbsp. Applesauce
1/2 cup peanut butter
1/3 cup powdered sugar
1 tbsp. butter
1/2 cup peanuts
2 tbsp. maple syrup

Directions:
Preheat oven to 350°F.
Place liners in a 12-muffin tin.
In a bowl, mix flour, salt, cinnamon and baking soda. Place aside
Using a bowl, beat the butter and sugars, until fluffy texture.

Add the egg, vanilla extract, and mashed bananas. Whisk until combined.
In another bowl, mix powdered sugar with peanut butter. Mix until smooth.
Spoon 1 tbsp. of the mixture into each muffin cup. Top each muffin with mixed melted butter with chopped peanuts and maple syrup.
Bake for 20-25 minutes. Let cool for 10 minutes before transferring to a cooling rack.

Nutrition:
Calories: 187 kcal
Protein: 8.12 g
Fat: 6.25 g
Carbohydrates: 27.82 g

27. Breakfast Pitas
Prep Time: 4 minutes
Cook Time: 6 minutes
Portions: 4

Ingredients:
1 tsp. onion powder
2 tsp. olive oil
1 tsp. garlic powder
8 egg whites
2 cup bell peppers
1 cup raw spinach
4 whole-wheat pita pockets

Directions:
Put the olive oil in a large sauté pan and place it over medium heat. When the oil is hot, toss in the chopped bell pepper and sauté for about 3 minutes or until tender. Add in the spinach now and sauté for about 1 to 3 minutes.
Place the egg whites into a small bowl, whisk well. Add in spices; whisk well. Pour the egg mixture into the sauté pan and scramble everything together.
Remove from heat and stuff 1/2 to 1 cup mixture into a pita pocket and serve.

Nutrition:
Calories: 153 kcal
Protein: 12.4 g
Fat: 3.41 g
Carbohydrates: 19.32 g

28. Pancakes with Berries
Prep Time: 5 minutes
Cook Time: 20 minutes
Portions: 2
Ingredients:
Pancake:

1 egg
1/4 cup spelled flour
1/4 cup almond flour
3 1/2 tsp. coconut flour
5 oz. water
salt
Filling:
1/3 cup mixed berries
3 tsp. chocolate
1 1/2 tsp. powdered sugar
4 tbsp. yogurt

Directions:

Put the flour, egg, and some salt in a bowl. Add the water. Mix everything with a whisk until a batter-like texture

Heat a coated pan. Put in half of the batter. Once the pancake is firm, turn it over. Take out the pancake, add the second half of the batter to the pan, and repeat. Melt chocolate over a water bath.

Let the pancakes cool. Brush the pancakes with the yogurt. Wash the berry and let it drain. Put berries on the yogurt. Roll up the pancakes.

Sprinkle them with powdered sugar.

Decorate the whole thing with the melted chocolate.

Nutrition:

Calories: 298 kcal Protein: 21 g
Fat: 9 g
Carbohydrates: 26 g

29. Simple Omelet

Prep Time: 10 minutes
Cook Time: 20 minutes
Portions: 2

Ingredients:

3 eggs
1/4 cup parmesan cheese
2 tbsp. heavy cream
1 tbsp. olive oil
1 tsp. oregano
nutmeg
salt
pepper
For covering:
3 - 4 stalks of basil
1 tomato
1/2 cup grated mozzarella

Directions:

Mix the cream and eggs in a medium bowl.
Add the grated parmesan, nutmeg, oregano, pepper and salt, and stir everything.

Heat the oil in a pan.
Add 1/2 of the egg and cream to the pan.
Let the omelet set over medium heat, turn it, and then remove it.
Repeat with the second half of the egg mixture.
Cut the tomatoes into slices and place them on top of the omelets.
Scatter the mozzarella over the tomatoes.
Place the omelets on a baking sheet.
Cook at 180°F for 5 to 10 minutes.
Then take the omelets out and decorate them with the basil leaves.

Nutrition:

Calories: 402 kcal
Protein: 21 g
Fat: 34 g
Carbohydrates: 7 g

30. Omelet with Tomatoes and Spring Onions

Prep Time: 5 minutes
Cook Time: 20 minutes
Portions: 2

Ingredients:

6 eggs
2 tomatoes
2 spring onions
1 shallot
2 tbsp. butter
1 tbsp. olive oil
1 pinch of nutmeg
Sea salt
Black pepper

Directions:

Whisk the eggs in a bowl.
Mix them and season with salt and pepper.
Peel the shallot and chop it up.
Clean the onions and cut them into rings.
Wash the tomatoes and cut them into pieces.
Heat butter and oil in a pan.
Braise half of the shallots in it.
Add half the egg mixture.
Let everything set over medium heat.
Scatter a few tomatoes and onion rings on top.
Repeat with the second half of the egg mixture.
In the end, spread the grated nutmeg over the whole thing.

Nutrition:

Calories: 263 kcal
Protein: 20.3 g

Fat: 24 g
Carbohydrates: 8 g

31. Pudding with Chia and Berries

Prep Time: 20 minutes
Cook Time: 45 minutes
Portions: 2
Ingredients:
1 cup raspberries and blueberries
1/4 cup chia seeds
17 oz. coconut milk
1 tsp. agave syrup
1/2 tsp. ground bourbon vanilla
Directions:
Put the chia seeds, agave syrup, and vanilla in a bowl.
Pour in the coconut milk.
Mix thoroughly and let it soak for 30 minutes.
Meanwhile, wash the berries and let them drain well.
Divide the coconut chia pudding between two glasses.
Put the berries on top.
Nutrition:
Calories: 662 kcal
Protein: 8 g
Fat: 55 g
Carbohydrates: 18 g

32. Scrambled Eggs with Eel and Bread

Prep Time: 5 minutes
Cook Time: 10 minutes
Portions: 2
Ingredients:
2 cup smoked eel
1 shallot
2 sticks of dill
4 slices of low carb bread
1 tbsp. oil
4 eggs
salt
pepper
Directions:
Mix the eggs in a bowl and season with salt and pepper.
Peel the shallot and cut it into fine cubes.
Chop the dill.
Remove the skin from the eel and cut it into pieces.
Heat the oil in a pan and steam the shallot in it.
Add the eggs and let them set.
Use the spatula to turn the eggs several times.
Reduce the heat and add the dill.

Stir everything.
Spread the scrambled eggs over four slices of bread.
Put the eel pieces on top.
Add some fresh dill and serve everything.
Nutrition:
Calories: 830 kcal
Protein: 45 g
Fat: 64 g
Carbohydrates: 8 g

33. Pomegranate, Nuts and Chia

Prep Time: 5 minutes
Cook Time: 10 minutes
Portions: 3
Ingredients:
1/4 cup hazelnuts
1/4 cup walnuts
1/2 cup almond milk
4 tbsp. chia seeds
4 tbsp. pomegranate seeds
1 tsp. agave syrup
Lime juice
Directions:
Finely chop the nuts.
Mix the almond milk with the chia seeds.
Let everything soak for 10 to 20 minutes.
Occasionally stir the mixture with the chia seeds.
Stir in the agave syrup.
Pour 2 tbsp. of each mixture into a dessert glass.
Layer the chopped nuts on top.
Cover the nuts with 1 tbsp. each of the chia mass.
Sprinkle the pomegranate seeds on top and serve everything.
Nutrition:
Calories: 248 kcal
Protein: 1 g
Fat: 19 g
Carbohydrates: 7 g

34. Blueberry Chia Seed Pudding

Prep Time: 1 hour 10 minutes
Cook Time: 0 minutes
Portions: 4
Ingredients:
1 cup blueberries
1/2 cup organic quark
1/2 cup soy yogurt
2 tbsp. hazelnuts
6 oz. almond milk
2 tbsp. chia seeds

2 tsp. agave syrup
2 tsp. of lavender
Directions:
Bring the almond milk to a boil along with the lavender. Let the mixture simmer for 10 minutes at a reduced temperature. Let them cool down afterward. If the milk is cold, add the blueberries and puree everything. Mix the whole thing with the chia seeds and agave syrup. Let everything soak in the refrigerator for an hour. Mix the yogurt and curd cheese. Add both to the crowd.
Divide the pudding into glasses.
Finely chop the hazelnuts and sprinkle them on top.
Nutrition:
Calories: 252 kcal
Protein: 1 g
Fat: 11 g
Carbohydrates: 12g

35. Oatmeal Yogurt
Prep Time: 5 minutes
Cook Time: 5 minutes
Portions: 1
Ingredients:
2/3 cup Greek-style yogurt
5 tsp. oatmeal
1/2 cup fresh persimmon
6 tsp. water
Directions:
Put the oatmeal in the pan.
Toast them, stirring constantly, until golden brown.
Then put them on a plate and let them cool down briefly.
Peel the persimmon and put it in a bowl with the water. Mix the whole thing into a fine puree.
Put the yogurt, the toasted oatmeal and then puree in layers in a glass and serve.
Nutrition:
Calories: 286 kcal
Protein: 1 g
Fat: 11 g
Carbohydrates: 29 g

36. Muesli Smoothie Bowl
Prep Time: 10 minutes
Cook Time: 0 minutes
Portions: 1
Ingredients:
2/3 cup yogurt
2 tbsp. apple

2 tbsp. mango
2 tbsp. low carb muesli
2 1/2 tsp. spinach
2 1/2 tsp. chia seeds
Directions:
Soak the spinach leaves and let them drain.
Peel the mango and cut it into strips.
Remove the apple core and cut it into pieces.
Put everything except the mango together with the yogurt in a blender and make a fine puree out of it.
Put the spinach smoothie in a bowl.
Add the muesli, chia seeds, and mango.
Serve the whole thing
Nutrition:
Calories: 362 kcal
Protein: 12 g
Fat: 21 g
Carbohydrates: 21 g

37. Fried Egg with Bacon
Prep Time: 5 minutes
Cook Time: 10 minutes
Portions: 1
Ingredients:
2 eggs
2 tbsp. of bacon
2 tbsp. olive oil
salt
pepper
Directions:
Heat oil in the pan and fry the bacon.
Reduce the heat and beat the eggs in the pan.
Cook the eggs and season with salt and pepper.
Serve the fried eggs hot with the bacon.
Nutrition:
Calories: 405 kcal
Protein: 19 g
Fat: 38 g
Carbohydrates: 1 g

38. Surprise Smoothie Bowl
Prep Time: 15 minutes
Cook Time: 0 minutes
Portions: 2
Ingredients:
1/4 banana
1 tsp. pumpkin seeds
5 tsp. blueberries
2 chopped walnuts
1 apple

1/4 cup raspberries
5 tsp. rolled oats
5 chopped almonds
2 1/2 tsp. poppy seeds
Agave syrup
1 1/4 cup yogurt

Directions:

Clean the fruit and let it drain.
Take some berries and set them aside.
Place the remaining berries in a tall mixing vessel.
Cut the banana into slices. Put a few aside.
Add the rest of the banana to the berries.
Remove the core of the apple and cut it into quarters.
Cut the quarters into thin wedges and set a few aside.
Add the remaining wedges to the berries.
Add the yogurt to the fruits and mix everything into a puree.
Sweeten the smoothie with the agave syrup.
Divide it into two bowls.
Serve it with the remaining fruit, poppy seeds, oatmeal, nuts, and seeds.

Nutrition:

Calories: 284 kcal Protein: 11 g
Fat: 19 g Carbohydrates: 21 g

39. Grain Bread and Avocado

Prep Time: 5 minutes
Cook Time: 0 minutes
Portions: 1

Ingredients:

1 stick of thyme
1/2 lime
1/2 cup of cottage cheese
1/2 avocado
2 slices of whole meal bread
chili flakes
salt
Black pepper

Directions:

Cut the avocado in half.
Remove the pulp and cut it into slices.
Pour the lime juice over it.
Wash the thyme and shake it dry.
Remove the leaves from the stem.
Brush the whole wheat bread with cottage cheese.
Place the avocado slices on top.
Top with chili flakes and thyme.
Add salt and pepper and serve.

Nutrition:

Calories: 490 kcal

Protein: 19 g Fat: 21 g
Carbohydrates: 31 g

40. Porridge with Walnuts

Prep Time: 5 minutes
Cook Time: 10 minutes
Portions: 1

Ingredients:

2 1/2 tsp. of oatmeal
1/2 cup blueberries
1/2 tsp. cinnamon
5 tsp. of crushed flaxseed
1/4 cup of ground walnuts
7 oz. nut drink
1/2 cup raspberries
agave syrup
salt

Directions:

Warm the nut drink in a small saucepan.
Add the walnuts, flaxseed, and oatmeal, stirring constantly.
Stir in the cinnamon and salt.
Simmer for 8 minutes.
Keep stirring everything.
Sweet the whole thing.
Put the porridge in a bowl.
Wash the berries and let them drain.
Add them to the porridge and serve everything.

Nutrition:

Calories: 378 kcal
Protein: 18 g
Fat: 27 g
Carbohydrates: 11 g

41. Peanut Butter Breakfast

Prep Time: 5 Minutes
Cook Time: 10 Minutes
Portions: 1

Ingredients:

1/3 cup quinoa flakes
chopped nuts
1/8 tsp. ground cinnamon
1/2 cup unsweetened nondairy milk
1 tbsp. natural creamy peanut butter
1 banana
1/2 cup of water
1/8 cup raw cacao powder
fresh berries

Directions:

Using an 8-quart pot over medium-high heat, stir together the quinoa flakes, milk, water, cacao powder, peanut butter, and cinnamon.

Cook and stir until the mixture begins to simmer.

Turn the heat to medium-low and cook for 3 to 5 minutes, stirring frequently.

Stir in the bananas and cook until hot.

Serve topped with fresh berries, nuts, and a splash of milk.

Nutrition:

Calories: 471 kcal

Protein: 18 g

Fat: 16 g

Carbohydrates: 69 g

42. Breakfast Cereal

Prep Time: 10 minutes

Cook Time: 3 minutes

Portions: 2

Ingredients:

4 tsp. ghee

1/3 cup walnuts; chopped.

1 tbsp. stevia

1/3 cup macadamia nuts; chopped.

1/3 cup flax seed

a pinch of salt

1/2 cup coconut; shredded

2 cup almond milk

Directions:

Heat a pot over medium heat. Add the milk, coconut, salt, macadamia nuts, walnuts, flax seeds, and stevia, and mix well.

Cook for 3 minutes. Stir again; remove from heat.

Let cool for 10 minutes

Divide into 2 bowls and serve

Nutrition:

Calories: 140 kcal

Protein: 7 g

Fat: 3 g

Carbohydrates: 1.5 g

43. Almond Coconut Cereal

Prep Time: 5 minutes

Cook Time: 5 minutes

Portions: 2

Ingredients:

2 tbsp. roasted sunflower seeds

1/2 cup blueberries

1/3 cup water

1 tbsp. chia seeds

1/3 cup coconut milk

2 tbsp. chopped almonds

Directions:

In a medium bowl add coconut milk and chia seeds; let it sit for 5 minutes.

Using a blender, pulse the almonds and the sunflower seeds.

Stir the combination to chia seeds mixture, and then add water to mix evenly.

Serve topped with the remaining sunflower seeds and blueberries

Nutrition:

Calories: 181 kcal

Protein: 3.7 g

Fat: 15.2 g

Carbohydrates: 10.8 g

44. Almond Porridge

Prep Time: 10 minutes

Cook Time: 5 minutes

Portions: 1

Ingredients:

1/4 tsp. ground cloves

1/4 tsp. nutmeg

1 tsp. stevia

3/4 cup coconut cream

1/2 cup ground almonds

1/4 tsp. ground cardamom

1 tsp. ground cinnamon

Directions:

Set a pan over medium heat to cook the coconut cream for a few minutes

Stir in almonds and stevia to cook for 5 minutes

Mix in nutmeg, cardamom, and cinnamon

Enjoy while still hot

Nutrition:

Calories: 695 kcal

Protein: 14.3 g

Fat: 66.7 g

Carbohydrates: 22 g

45. Bacon and Brussels Sprout Breakfast

Prep Time: 10 minutes

Cook Time: 15 minutes

Portions: 3

Ingredients:

1 1/2 tbsp. apple cider vinegar

salt

2 minced shallots
2 minced garlic cloves
3 medium eggs
12 oz. sliced Brussels sprouts
black pepper
2 oz. chopped bacon
1 tbsp. melted butter

Directions:
Over medium heat, quickly fry the bacon until crispy then reserve on a plate
Set the pan on fire again to fry garlic and shallots for 30 seconds
Stir in apple cider vinegar, Brussels sprouts, and seasoning to cook for five minutes
Add the bacon to cook for five minutes then stir in the butter and set a hole at the center
Crash the eggs to the pan and let cook fully
Enjoy!

Nutrition:
Calories: 275 kcal Protein: 17.4 g
Fat: 16.5 gCarbohydrates: 17. 2 g

46. Special Almond Cereal

Prep Time: 5 minutes
Cook Time: 5 minutes
Portions: 1

Ingredients:
2 tbsp. pepitas roasted
1/3 cup water
1/3 cup coconut milk
A handful blueberries
2 tbsp. almonds; chopped.
1 small banana; chopped.
1 tbsp. chia seeds

Directions:
In a bowl, mix chia seeds with coconut milk and leave aside for 5 minutes In your food processor, mix half of the pepitas with almonds and pulse them well. Add this to the chia seeds mix. Also, add the water and stir. Top with the rest of the pepitas, banana pieces, and blueberries, and serve

Nutrition:
Calories: 200 kcal Protein: 4 g
Fat: 3 g Carbohydrates: 5 g

47. Apple Cinnamon

Prep Time:
10 minutes
Cook Time: 8-9 hours
Portions:

4 minutes
Ingredients:
2 cup old-fashioned rolled oats
1 tsp. cinnamon
1/3 cup brown sugar
2 apples
4 cup water
pinch salt

Directions:
Peel and slice the apples and place them on the bottom of the slow cooker. Add brown sugar and cinnamon over the apples, and then stir until mixed. Pour the oats evenly over the apples and add water and salt. Cook on low for 8-9 hours (overnight). Stir well before serving, making sure to get the oats out of the bottom.

Nutrition:
Calories: 232.3 kcal Protein: 5.4 g Fat: 3.1 g
Carbohydrates: 53.2 g

48. Blueberry Moss Pancakes

Prep Time: 6 minutes
Cook Time: 20 minutes
Portions: 3

Ingredients:
2 tbsps. grape seed oil
1 cup coconut milk
1/2 cup blueberries
1/2 cup alkaline water
1/2 cup agave
2 cup spelt flour
1/4 tsp. sea moss

Directions:
Mix the spelt flour, agave, grape seed oil, hemp seeds, and sea moss in a bowl.
Add in 1 cup of hemp milk and alkaline water to the mixture until you get the consistent mixture you like.
Crimp the blueberries into the batter.
Heat the skillet to moderate heat, and then lightly coat it with the grape seed oil.
Pour the batter into the skillet, and then let them cook for approximately 5 minutes on every side.
Serve and Enjoy.

Nutrition:
Calories: 203 kcal Protein: 4.8 g
Fat: 1.4 g Carbohydrates: 41.6 g

49. Blueberry Moss Muffins

Prep Time: 5 Minutes
Cook Time: 20 minutes

Portions: 3
Ingredients:
1/2 cup blueberries
1 cup coconut milk
3/4 flour
grape seed oil
1/3 cup agave
1/4 cup sea moss gel
3/4 cup spelt flour
1/2 tsp. salt (preferable sea salt)
Directions:
Adjust the temperature of the oven to 365 °F.
Grease 6 regular-size muffin cups with muffin liners.
In a bowl, mix sea salt, sea moss, agave, coconut milk, and flour gel until they are properly blended.
You then crimp in blueberries.
Coat the muffin pan lightly with the grape seed oil.
Pour in the muffin batter.
Bake for at least 30 minutes until it turns golden brown.
Serve.
Nutrition:
Calories: 160.2 kcal
Proteins: 2.5 g
Fat: 5.1 g
Carbohydrates: 25.3 g

50. Crunchy Quinoa Meal

Prep Time: 5 minutes
Cook Time: 25 minutes
Portions: 2
Ingredients:
3 cup coconut milk
1/8 tsp. ground cinnamon
1 cup raspberry
1/2 cup chopped coconuts
1 cup rinsed quinoa
Directions:
In a saucepan, pour milk and bring to a boil over moderate heat.
Add the quinoa to the milk and then bring it to a boil once more.
You then let it simmer for at least 15 minutes on medium heat until the milk is reduced.
Stir in the cinnamon and mix properly.
Cover it, and then cook for 8 minutes until the milk is completely absorbed.
Add the raspberry and cook the meal for 30 seconds.
Serve and enjoy.
Nutrition:

Calories: 271 kcal
Protein: 6.5 g Fat: 3.7 g
Carbohydrates: 54.3 g

51. Coconut Pancakes

Prep Time: 5 minutes
Cook Time: 15 minutes
Portions: 4
Ingredients:
3 tbsp. coconut oil
1 cup coconut flour
2 tbsp. arrowroot powder
1 tsp. baking powder
1 cup coconut milk
2 tbsp. arrowroot powder
Directions:
In a medium container, mix in all the dry ingredients.
Add the coconut milk and 2 tbsps. of the coconut oil and mix properly.
In a skillet, melt 1 tsp. of coconut oil.
Pour a spoon of the batter into the skillet and spread evenly.
Cook it for like 3 minutes on medium heat until it becomes firm.
Turn the pancake to the other side, and then cook it for another 2 minutes until it turns golden brown.
Cook the remaining pancakes in the same process.
Serve.
Nutrition:
Calories: 377 kcal
Protein: 6.4 g
Fat: 14.9 g
Carbohydrates: 60.7 g

52. Quinoa Porridge

Prep Time: 5 minutes
Cook Time: 25 minutes
Portions: 2
Ingredients:
2 cup coconut milk
1 cup rinsed quinoa
1/8 tsp. ground cinnamon
1 cup fresh blueberries
Directions:
In a saucepan, boil the coconut milk over high heat.
Add the quinoa to the milk, and then bring the mixture to a boil.
Let it simmer for 15 minutes on medium heat until the milk is reduced.
Add the cinnamon, and then mix it properly in the saucepan.

Cover the saucepan and cook for at least 8 minutes until the milk is completely absorbed.

Add in the blueberries, and then cook for 30 more seconds.

Serve.

Nutrition:

Calories: 271 kcal Protein: 6.5 g

Fat: 3.7 g Carbohydrates: 54 g

53. Banana Barley Porridge

Prep Time: 15 minutes

Cook Time: 5 minutes

Portions: 2

Ingredients:

1 cup unsweetened coconut milk

1 small banana

1/2 cup barley

3 drops liquid stevia

1/4 cup chopped coconut

Directions:

In a bowl, properly mix barley with half of the coconut milk and stevia.

Cover the mixing bowl, then refrigerate for about 6 hours.

In a saucepan, mix the barley mixture with coconut milk.

Cook for about 5 minutes on moderate heat.

Then top it with the chopped coconuts and the banana slices.

Serve.

Nutrition:

Calories: 159 kcal

Protein: 4.6 g

Fat: 8.4 g

Carbohydrates: 19.8 g

54. Pumpkin Spice Quinoa

Prep Time: 10 minutes

Cook Time: 0 minutes

Portions: 2

Ingredients:

1 cup cooked quinoa

1 cup unsweetened coconut milk

1 large banana

1/4 cup pumpkin puree

1 tsp. pumpkin spice

2 tsp. chia seeds

Directions:

In a container, slice the banana and mix all the ingredients.

Shake the container with clod closed to mix well. Refrigerate overnight.

Serve.

Nutrition:

Calories: 212 kcal

Protein: 7.3 g

Fat: 11.9 g

Carbohydrates: 31.7 g

55. Tasty Breakfast Donuts

Prep Time: 5 minutes

Cook Time: 5 minutes

Portions: 4

Ingredients:

1 1/2 tbsp. coconut flour

5 drops Stevia (liquid form)

2 strips bacon

1/2 cup cream cheese

2 tbsp. erythritol

1/2 tsp. baking powder

1/2 tsp. vanilla extract

2 eggs

2 tbsp. almond flour

Directions:

Rub coconut oil over the donut maker and turn it on.

Mix all ingredients except bacon in a blender.

Pour batter into donut maker.

Leave for 3 minutes before flipping each donut.

Leave for another 2 minutes.

Take donuts out and let cool.

Crumble fried bacon into bits and use it to top donuts.

Nutrition:

Calories: 60 kcal

Protein: 3 g

Fat: 5 g

Carbohydrates: 1 g

56. Millet Porridge

Prep Time: 10 minutes

Cook Time: 20 minutes

Portions: 2

Ingredients:

1 tbsp. chopped coconut

3 drops liquid stevia

1/2 cup millet

1/2 cup unsweetened coconut milk

1 1/2 cup alkaline water

Sea salt

Directions:

Sauté the millet in a non-stick skillet for about 3 minutes.

Add salt and water and then stir.

Let the meal boil, and then reduce the amount of heat.

Cook for 15 minutes, and then add the remaining ingredients

Stir and cook the meal for 4 extra minutes.

Serve the meal with toping of the chopped nuts.

Nutrition:

Calories: 219 kcal

Protein: 6.4 g

Fat: 4.5 g

Carbohydrates: 38.2 g

57. Cream Cheese Egg Breakfast

Prep Time: 5 minutes

Cook Time: 5 minutes

Portions: 4

Ingredients:

2 eggs, beaten

1 tbsp. butter

2 tbsp. soft cream cheese with chives

Directions:

Melt the butter in a small skillet.

Add the eggs and cream cheese.

Stir and cook to desired doneness.

Nutrition:

Calories: 341 kcal Protein: 15 g

Fat: 31 g Carbohydrates: 0 g

58. Red Pepper Scrambled Eggs

Prep Time: 10 minutes

Cook Time: 12 minutes

Portions: 3

Ingredients:

2 eggs

1/2 tbsp. butter

1/2 avocado

1 1/2 roasted red pepper

Sea Salt

Directions:

In a nonstick skillet, heat the butter over medium heat. Break the eggs into the pan and break the yolks with a spoon. Sprinkle with a little salt.

Stir to stir and continue stirring until the eggs start to come out. Quickly add the bell peppers and avocado.

Cook and stir until the eggs suit your taste.

Nutrition:

Calories: 317 kcal

Protein: 14g Fat: 26 g

Carbohydrates: 4 g

59. Mushroom Quickie Scramble

Prep Time: 10 minutes

Cook Time: 10 minutes

Portions: 4

Ingredients:

1/2 cup of spinach

3 eggs

pepper

4 mushrooms

2 deli ham slices

1 tbsp. coconut oil

1/4 cup of red bell peppers

Salt

Directions:

Chop the ham and veggies.

Put half a tbsp. of butter in a frying pan and heat until melted.

Sauté the ham and vegetables in a frying pan then set aside.

Get a new frying pan and heat the remaining butter.

Add the whisked eggs into the second pan while stirring continuously to avoid overcooking.

When the eggs are done, sprinkle with salt and pepper to taste.

Add the ham and veggies to the pan with the eggs.

Mix well. Remove from burner and transfer to a plate.

Nutrition:

Calories: 350 kcal

Protein: 21.2 g

Fat: 29.9 g

Carbohydrates: 5.1 g

60. Coconut Coffee

Prep Time: 10 minutes

Cook Time: 10 minutes

Portions: 5

Ingredients:

2 cups of coffee

1 tbsp. of coconut milk

1/2 tbsp. of coconut oil

1/2 tbsp. of ghee

Directions:

Place the almond (or coconut) milk, coconut oil, ghee, and coffee in a blender Mix for around 10 seconds or until the coffee turns creamy and foamy. Pour contents into a coffee cup. Serve immediately and enjoy.

Nutrition:

Calories: 150 kcal Protein: 0g
Fat: 15.2 g Carbohydrates: 0 g

61. Tasty Veggie Waffles

Prep Time: 10 minutes
Cook Time: 9 minutes
Portions: 3

Ingredients:

3 cup raw cauliflower
1 cup cheddar cheese
1 cup mozzarella cheese
1/2 cup parmesan
1/3 cup chives
6 eggs
1 tsp. garlic powder
1 tsp. onion powder
1/2 tsp. chili flakes
Salt
Black pepper

Directions:

Turn the waffle maker on.

Grate the cauliflower. Finely slice the chives. In a bowl, mix all the listed ingredients very well until incorporated. Once the waffle maker is hot, distribute the waffle mixture into the insert. Let cook for about 9 minutes, flipping at 6 minutes. Remove from waffle maker and set aside. Serve and enjoy!

Nutrition:

Calories: 390 kcal
Protein: 30 g
Fat: 28 g
Carbohydrates: 6 g

62. Omega 3 Breakfast Shake

Prep Time: 5 minutes
Cook Time: 5 minutes
Portions: 2

Ingredients:

1 cup vanilla almond milk
2 tbsp. blueberries
1 1/2 tbsp. flaxseed meal
1 tbsp. Oil
3/4 tbsp. banana extract
1/2 tbsp. chia seeds
5 drops Stevia
1/8 tbsp. Xanthan gum

D i rections:

In a blender, mix vanilla almond milk, banana extract, Stevia, and three ice cubes.

When smooth, add blueberries and pulse.

Once blueberries are thoroughly incorporated, add flaxseed meal and chia seeds.

Let sit for 5 minutes.

After 5 minutes, pulse again until all ingredients are nicely distributed. Serve and enjoy

Nutrition:

Calories: 264 kcal
Protein: 4 g Fat: 25 g
Carbohydrates: 7 g

63. Muffins with Bacon and Thyme

Prep Time: 10 minutes
Cook Time: 20 minutes
Portions: 3

Ingredients:

1/2 cup of melted ghee
4 eggs
2 tsp. of lemon thyme
1 cup bacon bits
1 tsp. of baking soda
3 cups of almond flour
Sea salt

Directions:

Preheat oven to 350°F.

Put ghee in the mixing bowl and melt.

Add baking soda and almond flour.

Put the eggs in.

Add the lemon thyme (if preferred, other herbs or spices may be used).

Drizzle with salt.

Mix all ingredients well.

Sprinkle with bacon bits

Line the muffin pan with liners.

Spoon mixture into the pan, filling the pan to about 3/4 full.

Bake for about 20 minutes. Test by inserting a toothpick into a muffin. If it comes out clean, then the muffins are done.

Nutrition:

Calories: 300 kcal
Protein: 11 g
Fat: 28 g
Carbohydrates: 6 g

64. Amaranth Porridge

Prep Time: 5 minutes
Cook Time: 30 minutes
Portions: 2

Ingredients:

1 cup amaranth

2 tbsps. coconut oil
2 cup coconut milk
1 tbsp. ground cinnamon
2 cup alkaline water

Directions:

In a saucepan, mix the milk with water, and then boil the mixture.

Cook on medium heat, and then simmer for at least 30 minutes as you stir it occasionally.

Turn off the heat.

Add in cinnamon and coconut oil and then stir.

Serve.

Nutrition:

Calories: 434 kcal

Protein: 6.7 g

Fat: 35 g

Carbohydrates: 27 g

65. Gluten-Free Pancakes

Prep Time: 5 minutes

Cook Time: 2 minutes

Portions: 2

Ingredients:

1 cup low-fat cream cheese
1 scoop protein powder
1/4 cup almond meal
1 1/12 tsp. baking powder
1 cup low-fat cream cheese
6 eggs
Sea salt

Directions:

Combine dry ingredients in a blender. Add the eggs one after another and then the cream cheese. Mix well.

Lightly grease a skillet with Cooking spray and place over medium-high heat.

Pour the batter into the pan. Turn the pan gently to create round pancakes.

Cook for about 2 minutes on each side.

Serve pancakes with your favorite topping.

Nutrition:

Calories: 288 kcal

Protein: 25 g

Fat: 14 g

Carbohydrates: 5 g

66. Mushroom & Spinach Omelet

Prep Time: 20 minutes

Cook Time: 20 minutes

Portions: 3

Ingredients:

2 tbsp. butter
6-8 (5 oz.) mushrooms
salt
pepper
1/2 oz. baby spinach
garlic powder
4 eggs
1 oz. shredded Swiss cheese

Directions:

In a very large saucepan, sauté the sliced mushrooms in one tbsp. of butter until soft. Season with salt, pepper, and garlic. Remove the mushrooms from the pan and keep warm. Heat the remaining tbsp. of butter in the same skillet over medium heat.

Beat the eggs with a little salt and pepper and add to the hot butter. Turn the pan over to coat the entire bottom of the pan with an egg. Once the egg is almost out, place the cheese over the middle of the tortilla. Fill the cheese with spinach leaves and hot mushrooms. Let cook for about a minute for the spinach to start to wilt. Fold the empty side of the tortilla carefully over the filling and slide it onto a plate and sprinkle with chives, if desired.

Alternatively, you can make two tortillas using half the mushroom, spinach, and cheese filling in each.

Nutrition:

Calories: 321 kcal

Protein: 19 g

Fat: 26 g

Carbohydrates: 4 g

67. Sweet Cashew Cheese Spread

Prep Time: 5 minutes

Cook Time: 5 minutes

Portions: 10 Portions

Ingredients:

5 drops stevia
2 cup cashews
1/2 cup water

Directions:

Soak the cashews overnight in water.

Next, drain the excess water then transfer cashews to a food processor. Add in the stevia and the water. Process until smooth.

Serve chilled. Enjoy.

Nutrition:

Calories: 31 kcal

Protein: 1.03 g

Fat: 2.49 g
Carbohydrates: 1.71 g

68. Whole-Wheat Blueberry Muffins

Prep Time: 5 minutes
Cook Time: 25 minutes
Portions: 8
Ingredients:
1 tsp. vanilla extract
1/2 cup milk
1/2 cup maple syrup
2 cup whole-wheat flour
1/2 tsp. baking soda
1/2 cup unsweetened applesauce
1 cup blueberries
Directions:
Preheat the oven to 375°F.
In a large bowl, mix the milk, applesauce, maple syrup, and vanilla.
Stir in the flour and baking soda until no dry flour is left and the batter is smooth.
Gently fold in the blueberries until they are evenly distributed throughout the batter.
In a muffin tin, fill eight muffin cups with three-quarters full of batter.
Bake for 25 minutes, or until you can stick a knife into the center of a muffin and it comes out clean. Allow cooling before serving.
Nutrition:
Calories: 209 kcal
Protein: 3.95 g
Fat: 0.94 g
Carbohydrates: 46.55 g

69. Hemp Seed Porridge

Prep Time: 5 minutes
Cook Time: 5 minutes
Portions: 6
Ingredients:
3 cup cooked hemp seed
1 pack stevia
1 cup coconut milk
Directions:
In a saucepan, cook the rice and coconut milk over medium heat, stirring constantly, for about 5 minutes. Remove the pot from the heat, and then add the stevia. Stir.
Serve in 6 bowls.

Nutrition:
Calories: 236 kcal
Protein: 7 g
Fat: 1.8 g
Carbohydrates: 48.3 g

70. Walnut Crunch Banana Bread

Prep Time: 5 minutes
Cook Time: 1 hour and 30 minutes
Portions: 1
Ingredients:
1/2 tsp. baking soda
1/4 cup maple syrup
1 tsp. vanilla extract
1 1/2 cup whole-wheat flour
1/2 tsp. ground cinnamon
4 ripe bananas
1/4 cup walnut pieces
1 tbsp. apple cider vinegar
Directions:
Preheat the oven to 350°F.
In a large bowl, mash bananas with a fork until they have a mashed consistency. Stir in the maple syrup, apple cider vinegar, and vanilla. Stir in the flour, cinnamon, and baking soda. Fold in the walnut pieces.
Carefully pour the batter into a loaf pan. Bake for 1 hour, or until you can pierce the center with a knife, and it comes out clean.
Remove the cake from the oven and let it cool on the countertop for at least 30 minutes before serving.
Nutrition:
Calories: 655 kcal
Protein: 12.27 g
Fat: 1.72 g
Carbohydrates: 151.93 g

Chapter 3:

Lunch Recipes

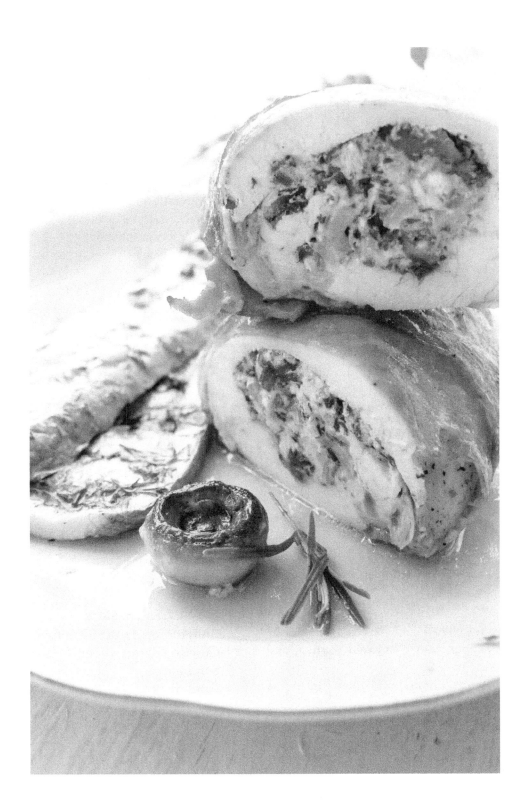

71. Spinach Chicken

Preparation Time: 10 minutes
Cooking Time: 10 minutes
Servings: 2
Ingredients:
2 garlic cloves, minced
2 tablespoons unsalted butter, divided
¼ cup parmesan cheese, shredded
¾ pound chicken tenders
¼ cup heavy cream
10 ounces frozen spinach, chopped
Salt and black pepper, to taste
Directions:
Heat 1 tablespoon of butter in a large skillet and add chicken, salt, and black pepper.
Cook for about 3 minutes on both sides and pass the chicken to a bowl.
Melt the remaining butter in the skillet and add garlic, cheese, heavy cream, and spinach.
Cook for about 2 minutes and add the chicken.
Cook for about 5 minutes on low heat and dish out to immediately serve.
Place chicken in a dish and set aside to cool for meal prepping. Divide it into 2 containers and cover them. Refrigerate for about 3 days and reheat in microwave before serving.
Nutrition: Calories: 288 Carbs: 3.6g Protein: 27.7g Fat: 18.3g Sugar: 0.3g

72. Lemongrass Prawns

Preparation Time: 10 minutes
Cooking Time: 15 minutes
Servings: 2
Ingredients:
½ red chili pepper, seeded and chopped
2 lemongrass stalks
½ pound prawns, deveined and peeled
6 tablespoons butter
¼ teaspoon smoked paprika
Directions:
Preheat the oven to 390°F and grease a baking dish.
Mix red chili pepper, butter, smoked paprika, and prawns in a bowl.
Marinate for about 2 hours, and then thread the prawns on the lemongrass stalks.
Arrange the threaded prawns on the baking dish and transfer them to the oven.
Bake for about 15 minutes and dish out to serve immediately.

Place the prawns in a dish and set them aside to cool for meal prepping. Divide it into 2 containers and close the lid. Refrigerate for about 4 days and reheat in microwave before serving.
Nutrition: Calories: 322 Carbs: 3.8g Protein: 34.8g Fat: 18g Sugar: 0.1g Sodium: 478mg

73. Honey Glazed Chicken Drumsticks

Preparation Time: 10 minutes
Cooking Time: 20 minutes
Servings: 2
Ingredients:
½ tablespoon fresh thyme, minced
1/8 cup Dijon mustard
½ tablespoon fresh rosemary, minced
½ tablespoon honey
2 chicken drumsticks
1 tablespoon olive oil
Salt and black pepper, to taste
Directions:
Preheat the oven at 325°F and grease a baking dish.
Combine all the ingredients in a bowl except the drumsticks and mix well.
Add drumsticks and coat generously with the mixture.
Cover and refrigerate to marinate overnight.
Place the drumsticks in the baking dish and transfer them to the oven.
Cook for about 20 minutes and dish out to immediately serve.
Place chicken drumsticks in a dish and set them aside to cool for meal prepping.
Divide it into 2 containers and cover them. Refrigerate for about 3 days and reheat in microwave before serving.
Nutrition: Calories: 301 Carbs: 6g Fat: 19.7g Proteins: 4.5g Sugar: 4.5g Sodium: 316mg

74. Crab Cakes

Preparation Time: 20 minutes
Cooking Time: 10 minutes
Servings: 2
Ingredients:
½ pound lump crabmeat, drained
2 tablespoons coconut flour
1 tablespoon mayonnaise
¼ teaspoon green Tabasco sauce
3 tablespoons butter
1 small egg, beaten

¾ tablespoon fresh parsley, chopped
½ teaspoon yellow mustard
Salt and black pepper, to taste
Directions:
Mix all the ingredients in a bowl except butter.
Make patties from this mixture and set them aside.
Heat butter in a skillet over medium heat and add patties.
Cook for about 10 minutes on each side and dish out to serve hot.
You can store the raw patties in the freezer for about 3 weeks for meal prepping. Place patties in a container and place parchment paper in between the patties to avoid stickiness.
Nutrition: Calories: 153 Fat: 10.8g Carbs: 6.7g Protein: 6.4g Sugar: 2.4 Sodium: 46mg

75. Flavorful Taco Soup

Preparation Time: 5 minutes
Cooking Time: 15
Servings: 8
Ingredients:
1 pound ground beef
3 tablespoons taco seasoning, divided
4 cups beef bone broth
2 14.5-oz cans diced tomatoes
3/4 cup Ranch dressing
Directions:
Put the ground beef into a pot and place over medium-high heat, and cook until brown, about 10 minutes.
Add in ¾ cup of broth and two tablespoons of taco seasoning. Cook until part of the liquid has evaporated. Add in the diced tomatoes, the rest of the broth, and the rest of the taco seasoning. Stir to mix, then simmer for ten minutes. Remove the pot from heat and add in the ranch dressing. Garnish with cilantro and cheddar cheese. Serve.
Nutrition: Calories: 309 Fat: 24g Protein: 13g

76. Delicious Instant Pot Buffalo Chicken Soup

Preparation Time: 10 minutes
Cooking Time: 20 minutes
Servings: 6
Ingredients:
1 tablespoon Olive oil
½ Onion, diced)
½ cup Celery, diced
4 cloves Garlic, minced
1 pound Shredded chicken, cooked
4 cups chicken bone broth, or any chicken broth
3 tablespoons Buffalo sauce
6 ounces Cream cheese
1/2 cup Half & half
Directions:
Switch the instant pot to the sauté function. Add in the chopped onion, oil, and celery. Cook until the onions are brown and translucent, about 10 minutes. Add in the garlic and cook until fragrant, about 1 minute. Switch off the instant pot.
Add in the broth, shredded chicken, and buffalo sauce. Cover the instant pot and seal. Switch the soup feature on and set the time to 5 minutes.
When cooked, release pressure naturally for 5 minutes and then quickly.
Scoop out one cup of the soup liquid into a blender bowl, then add in the cheese and blend until smooth. Pour the puree into the instant pot, then add in the half and half and stir to mix.
Serve.
Nutrition: Servings: 1 cup Calories: 270 Protein: 27g Fat: 16g Carbohydrates: 4g

77. Chicken Curry

Preparation Time: 10 minutes
Cooking Time: 30 minutes
Servings: 2
Ingredients:
2 chicken breasts
1 garlic clove
1 small onion
1 zucchini
2 carrots
1 box bamboo shoots or sprouts
1 cup coconut milk
1 tablespoon tomato paste
2 tablespoons yellow curry paste
Directions:
Mince the onion and sauté in a pan with a little oil for a few minutes.
Add chicken cut in large cubes and crushed garlic, salt, pepper and sauté quickly over high heat until meat begins to color.
Pour zucchini and carrots in thick slices into the pan. Sear over high heat for a few minutes, then add the coconut milk, tomato sauce, bamboo shoots, and 1 to 2 tablespoons curry paste, depending on your taste. Cook over low heat and cover for 30 to 45 minutes, stirring occasionally

Once cooked, divide the chicken curry between 2 containers
Store the containers in the refrigerator
Nutrition: Calories: 626 Fat: 53.2 g Carbs: 9 g Protein: 27.8 g Sugar: 3 g;

78. Chicken and Broccoli Gratin

Preparation Time: 10 minutes,
Cooking Time: 10 minutes
Servings: 2
Ingredients:
1 pound chicken breasts
1/4 cup almond butter
100 cl fresh cream
1 cup goat cheese
2 organic eggs
2 Crushed garlic cloves
1 pinch salt
1 pinch pepper
Directions:
Cook the broccoli in a pot of water for 10 minutes. It must remain firm.
Melt the butter in a skillet; add the crushed garlic clove and the salted and peppered chicken. Let it get a brown color.
Drain the broccoli and mix with the chicken.
Beat the eggs with cream, salt, and pepper. Place broccoli and chicken in a baking dish, cover with cream mixture and sprinkle with grated cheese.
Put in the oven at 390°F for 20 minutes.
When the gratin is ready; set it aside to cool for 3 minutes
Cut the gratin into 2 halves or in 4 portions
Place every 2 portions of gratin in a container so that you have two containers.
Nutrition: Calories: 612 Fat: 48 g Carbs: 11 g Protein: 34 g Sugar: 1 g

79. Shrimp Salad Cocktails

Preparation Time: 35 minutes
Cooking Time: 35 minutes
Servings: 8 servings
Ingredients:
2 cups mayonnaise
6 plum tomatoes, seeded and finely chopped
¼ cup ketchup
¼ cup lemon juice
2 cups seedless red and green grapes, halved
1 tablespoon Worcestershire sauce
2 pound peeled and deveined cooked large shrimp
2 celery ribs, finely chopped
3 tablespoons minced fresh tarragon or 3 teaspoons dried tarragon
1/4 teaspoon Salt and pepper
2 cups romaine Shredded
1/2 cup Papaya or peeled chopped mango
Parsley or minced chives
Directions:
Combine Worcestershire sauce, lemon juice, ketchup, and mayonnaise in a small bowl. Combine pepper, salt, tarragon, celery, and shrimp together in a large bowl. Put in 1 cup of dressing, toss well to coat.
Scoop 1 tablespoon of the dressing into 8 cocktail glasses. Layer each glass with 1/4 cup of lettuce, followed by 1/2 cup of the shrimp mixture, 1/4 cup of grapes, 1/3 cup of tomatoes, and finally 1 tablespoon of mango. Spread the remaining dressing over top; sprinkle chives on top. Serve immediately.
Nutrition: Calories: 580 Total Carbohydrate: 16 g Cholesterol: 192 mg Total Fat: 46 g Fiber: 2 g Protein: 24 g

80. Beet Greens with Pine Nuts Goat Cheese

Preparation Time: 25 minutes
Cooking Time: 15 minutes
Servings: 3
Ingredients:
4 cups beet tops, washed and chopped roughly
1 teaspoon EVOO
1 tablespoon no sugar added balsamic vinegar
2 ounces crumbled dry goat cheese
2 tablespoons toasted pine nuts
Directions:
Warm the oil in a pan, then cook the beet greens on medium-high heat until they release their moisture. Let it cook until almost tender. Flavor with salt and pepper and remove from heat. Toss the greens in a mixture of balsamic vinegar and olive oil, then top with the nuts and cheese. Serve warm.
Nutrition: Calories: 215 Total Carbohydrate: 4 g Cholesterol: 12 mg Total Fat: 18 g Fiber: 2 g Protein: 10 g

81. Shrimp with Dipping Sauce

Preparation Time: 5 minutes
Cooking Time: 15 minutes
Servings: 6
Ingredients:
1 tablespoon reduced-sodium soy sauce

2 teaspoons Hot pepper sauce
1 teaspoon canola oil
¼ teaspoon garlic powder
1/8 to ¼ teaspoon cayenne pepper
1 pound uncooked medium shrimp, peeled and deveined
2 tablespoons chopped green onions
Dipping Sauce:
3 tablespoons Reduced-sodium soy sauce
1 teaspoon rice vinegar
1 tablespoon orange juice
2 teaspoons Sesame oil
2 teaspoons Honey
1 garlic clove, minced
1 ½ teaspoons Minced fresh ginger root

Directions:
Heat the initial 5 ingredients in a big nonstick frying pan for 30 seconds, then mix continuously.
Add onions and shrimp, and stir fry for 4–5 minutes or until the shrimp turns pink.
Mix together the sauce and serve it with the shrimp.
Nutrition: Calories: 97 Total Carbohydrate: 4 g Cholesterol: 112 mg Total Fat: 3 g Fiber: 0 g Protein: 13 g

82. Shrimp, Mushroom, And Broccoli
Preparation Time: 15 minutes
Cooking Time: 8 minutes
Servings: 2
Ingredients:
1 pound shrimp
2 garlic, minced
1 cup broccoli
2 tablespoons soy sauce
1 teaspoon stevia
Oil spray, for greasing
1 tablespoon lemon juice
½ pound shitake mushroom

Directions:
Preheat the air fryer by selecting air fry mode for 5 minutes at 350°F. Select start/pause to begin the preheating process. Once preheating is done, press start/pause. Take a bowl and add the shrimp, minced garlic, soy sauce, and stevia. Then, add lemon juice and vegetables. Toss all the ingredients well
Add it to the air fryer basket that is greased with oil spray.
Set it to air fry mode at 390°F, for 8 minutes.
Once done, take out the ingredients and serve.
Serving Suggestion: Serve it with mashed potatoes

Variation Tip: Use coconut amino instead of soy sauce.
Nutritional Information Per Serving: Calories: 259 | Fat: 4.6g| Sodium: 1744mg | Carbs: 23.5g | Fiber: 3.7g | Sugar: 5.3g | Protein: 55.8g

83. Lemon Tilapia Parmesan
Preparation Time: 12 minutes
Cooking Time: 15 minutes
Servings: 3
Ingredients:
1 ½ pound of tilapia fillet or codfish fillet
2 tablespoons olive oil
2 cloves garlic, minced
Salt and ground black pepper
2 cayenne pepper dashes
1 ½ tablespoon lemon juice
½ cup Parmesan cheese, shredded

Directions:
Pat dries the tilapia fillet with a paper towel and season it with, cayenne pepper, lemon juice, minced garlic, olive oil, salt, and black pepper.
Grease the air fryer basket with oil spray.
Put the fish in the air fryer basket.
Insert the basket into the unit.
Use AIRFRY mode at 350°F for 15 minutes.
Once done, serve by topping it with cheese.
Serving Suggestion: Serve with lime wedges
Variation Tip: Use hard cheese for sprinkling.
Low Nutrition Per Serving: Calories: 414| Fat: 17.5g| Sodium: 15064mg | Carbs: 1.9g | Fiber: 0.1g | Sugar: 0.2g | Protein: 68.9g

84. Steak and Cabbage
Preparation Time: 25 minutes
Cooking Time: 20 minutes
Servings: 4
Ingredients:
1 pound sirloin steak, sliced
4 tablespoons of peanut oil
2 cups cabbage
2 green bell pepper
2 onions, chopped
2 cloves garlic, sliced
Salt and black pepper, to taste

Directions:
Preheat the air fryer to 400°F for 10 minutes.
Rub the steak with half of the peanut oil, salt, and black pepper, and set aside.
Take a bowl, add oil and cabbage.

Put the cabbage in the air fryer basket and air fry for 4 minutes.

Take out the cabbage.

Afterward, add the steak, bell pepper, garlic cloves, and onions.

Air fry for 15 minutes.

Remember to flip halfway through.

Once done, serve.

Serving Suggestion: Serve with French fries

Variation Tip: None

Nutritional Information Per Serving: Calories: 363 | Fat: 20.7g | Sodium: 83mg | Carbs: 7.7g | Fiber: 2.1g | Sugar: 3.5g | Protein: 35.6g

85. Beef Patties

Preparation Time: 22 minutes
Cooking Time: 18 minutes
Servings: 5
Ingredients:

1.5 pounds beef, grounded

Salt and black pepper, to taste

2 tablespoons olive oil

1 cup white onions, chopped

2 green peppers, chopped

¼ teaspoon coriander powder

¼ teaspoon turmeric

½ teaspoon cumin, grounded

2 large tomatoes, chopped or sliced

2 onions, chopped

Oil spray, for greasing

Directions:

Combine all the listed ingredients in a bowl and make patties by hand.

Grease the patties with oil spray from both sides.

Arrange it inside the air fryer basket.

Air fry at 400°F for 18 minutes.

Remember to flip halfway through.

Serve.

Serving Suggestion: Serve with salad

Variation Tip: None

Nutritional Information Per Serving: Calories: 332 | Fat: 14.3g | Sodium 92mg | Carbs: 5.7g | Fiber: 1.3g | Sugar: 2.1g | Protein: 42.6g

86. Lean Beef

Preparation Time: 15 minutes
Cooking Time: 14 minutes
Servings: 4
Ingredients:

1 pound flank steak, lean

¼ cup tapioca starch

Sauce **Ingredients:**

2 teaspoons of vegetable oil

½ teaspoon of ginger garlic paste

1/3 cup coconut amino

1/3 cup water

¼ cup stevia

Directions:

Rub steak with corn starch and put it in a baking tray.

Air fryer for 4 minutes at 400°F.

In a cooking pan heat all the sauce ingredients.

Put the steak in the sauce and let it cook for 2 minutes per side.

Enjoy.

Serving Suggestion: Serve with Mashed Potatoes or cauliflower rice

Variation Tip: None

Nutritional Information Per Serving: Calories: 321 | Fat: 11.7g | Sodium 1264mg | Carbs: 19g | Fiber: 0.2g | Sugar: 9.2g | Protein: 32.9g

87. Lamb Chops with Yogurt

Preparation Time: 14 minutes
Cooking Time: 15 minutes
Servings: 6
Ingredients:

6 tablespoons Greek yogurt

1 teaspoon cumin seeds

¼ tablespoon coriander seeds, crushed

¼ teaspoon chili powder

½ teaspoon Gram Masala

2 tablespoons lemon juice

Salt, to taste

6 lamb chops

Oil spray for greasing

Directions:

Mix all the ingredients in a bowl and marinate the chops in it for 1 hour in the refrigerator.

Preheat air fryer to 400°F.

Then grease an air fryer basket and place chops on the basket.

Air fry the chops for 15 minutes.

Serve and enjoy.

Serving Suggestion: Serve with cauliflower rice

Variation Tip: None

Nutritional Information Per Serving: Calories: 662 | Fat: 25g | Sodium: 300mg | Carbs: 3g | Fiber: 0.1g | Sugar: 2.8g | Protein: 98g

88. Chicken and Spinach Quiche

Preparation Time: 15 minutes
Cooking Time: 12 minutes
Servings: 4
Ingredients:
4 eggs, whisked
1 cup spinach
½ cup cashew cream
3 tablespoons mustard
1 cup grated Swiss cheese
½ teaspoon thyme
1 cup chicken, cooked and shredded
Pinch salt and freshly ground black pepper
Directions:
Take a baking pan and grease it with oil spray.
Take a large bowl and all the listed ingredients.
Pour the mixture into the baking pan.
Add it to the air fryer basket.
Cook for 12 minutes at 400°F, in the air fryer.
Once the egg gets cooked, and cheese melts, serve.
Serving Suggestion: Serve with Cream cheese topping
Variation Tip: None
Nutritional Information Per Serving: Calories: 271| Fat: 16.2g| Sodium: 149mg | Carbs: 5.8g | Fiber: 1.5g | Sugar: 1.3g | Protein: 25.3g

89. Parmesan Crush Chicken

Preparation Time: 12 minutes
Cooking Time: 15 minutes
Servings: 2
Ingredients:
2 chicken breasts
½ cup parmesan cheese
2 eggs, whisked
Salt, to taste
Oil spray, for greasing
Directions:
Preheat the air fryer by selecting AIR FRY mode for 6 minutes at 350°F.
Select start/pause to begin the preheating process.
Once preheating is done, press start/pause.
Crack the egg in a small or medium bowl and set it aside.
Rub the chicken breast with salt and coat it with egg.
Next, dredge it in the parmesan cheese.
Cover the basket of the air fryer with parchment paper.
Arrange the breast pieces onto the basket, and grease the breasts with oil spray.

Set it to air fry mode at 375°F, for 15 minutes.
Once it's done, serve.
Serving Suggestion: Serve it with cauliflower rice
Variation Tip: None
Nutritional Information Per Serving: Calories: 314| Fat: 16.2g| Sodium: 503mg | Carbs: 1.8g | Fiber: 0g | Sugar: 0.3g | Protein: 40.2g

90. Chicken with Avocado Salsa

Preparation Time: 15 minutes
Cooking Time: 22 minutes
Servings: 6
Ingredients:
Chicken **Ingredients:**
2 pounds raw skinless chicken
1/3 cup cilantro, chopped
2 clove garlic
½ teaspoon Cumin
2 tablespoons lime juice
2 teaspoons vegetable oil
Salt and black pepper, to taste
Salsa **Ingredients:**
1 cup tomatoes, chopped
2 avocados, pitted and chopped
2 teaspoons red onion
1 teaspoon lime juice
Salt and black pepper, to taste
¼ teaspoon pepper
Directions:
Mix the cilantro, garlic, lime juice, salt, cumin, and vegetable oil in a bowl, and marinate the chicken in it by coating the chicken well with the mixture.
Preheat the air fryer for 10 minutes at 390°F
Afterward, bake the chicken in the air fryer at 390°F for 22 minutes. Remember to flip the chicken halfway through. Mix well all the salsa ingredients in a bowl and serve it with chicken.
Serving Suggestion: Serve with it steamed vegetables
Variation Tip: None
Nutritional Information Per Serving: Calories: 447| Fat: 25.9g| Sodium: 137mg | Carbs: 7.8g | Fiber: 5g | Sugar: 1.3g | Protein: 45.4g

91. Air Fryer Glazed Chicken and Vegetables

Preparation Time: 25 minutes
Cooking Time: 25 minutes
Servings: 4
Ingredients:
2 teaspoons Coconut Amino

½ teaspoon Worcestershire Sauce

2 teaspoons Stevie

1 teaspoon Ginger

1 teaspoon Garlic, Crushed

4 chicken Thighs

12 ounces Mixed green Vegetables

Directions:

Take a bowl and mix coconut amino, Worcestershire sauce, stevia, ginger, and garlic.

Add the chicken to it and let the chicken marinate for few hours.

Grease the basket of the air fryer with oil spray.

Slice the chicken into small pieces and arrange it in the basket along with the vegetables.

Coat with oil spray.

Air Fry for 25 minutes at 390°F.

Flipping halfway through.

Once done, serve.

Serving Suggestion: Serve it with salad

Variation Tip: use soy sauce instead of coconut amino

Nutritional Information Per Serving: Calories: 225| Fat: 10g| Sodium: 704mg | Carbs: 14g | Fiber: 1.9g | Sugar: 3g | Protein: 23.5g

92. Tilapia with Green Beans

Preparation Time: 15 minutes

Cooking Time: 12 minutes

Servings: 2

Ingredients:

2 tilapia fillets, 4 ounces each

2 teaspoons olive oil

2 teaspoons smoked paprika

Salt and black pepper, to taste

1 cup broccoli

2 tablespoons lemon juice

1 cup green beans

Oil spray, for greasing

Directions:

Grease the broccoli and green beans with oil spray, and season with salt and black pepper.

Rub the salmon fillet with olive oil, smoked paprika, salt, and lemon juice

Put the salmon fillets in the basket of the air fryer along with vegetables

Now set it to AIRFRY mode at 400°F for 12 minutes. Take out the basket after 7 minutes and transfer the vegetable to the serving plate.

Once the salmon is done, take out and serve with greens

Serving Suggestion: Serve with mashed potatoes

Variation Tip: None

Nutritional Information Per Serving: Calories: 517 | Fat: 1 3.2g| Sodium: 254mg | Carbs: 8.5g | Fiber: 3.9g | Sugar: 2.1g | Protein: 92.7g

93. Sundried Tomato Salmon

Preparation Time: 20 minutes

Cooking Time: 12 minutes

Servings: 2

Ingredients:

8 ounces raw salmon

¼ cup fresh parsley, chopped

2 tablespoons Sun-Dried Tomato Dressing

Oil spray, for greasing

Salt and black pepper, to taste

4 Cherry tomatoes

1 cup broccoli, florets

Directions:

First, preheat the air fryer to 350°F. Combine parsley, dressing, salt, and pepper in a bowl, and set aside.

Brush the salmon with a bowl mixture and grease it with oil spray. Put the salmon fillets in the basket of the air fryer along with vegetables.

Now set it to air fry mode at 400°F for 12 minutes.

Baste the salmon two times during cooking.

Once it's done, serve

Serving Suggestion: None

Variation Tip: None

Nutritional Information Per Serving: Calories: 275| Fat: 13g| Sodium: 231mg | Carbs: 18.1g | Fiber: 4.4g | Sugar: 11g | Protein: 25.7g

94. Thai Green Curry

Preparation Time: 15 minutes.

Cooking Time: 10 minutes.

Serving: 2

Ingredients:

Fish:

2 cod fillets

2 halibut fillets

2 snapper fillets

1 lemon

2 cups coconut milk

3 ounces baby spinach

2 ounces carrots, shredded

Directions:

Add coconut milk and the rest of the ingredients to a cooking pot.

Cook this mixture for 10 minutes on medium heat.

Serve warm.
Serving Suggestion: Serve the curry with white rice.
Variation Tip: Drizzle cheese on top for a rich taste.
Nutritional Information Per Serving: Calories: 351 | Fat: 4g |Sodium 236mg | Carbs: 19.1g | Fiber: 0.3g | Sugar: 0.1g | Protein: 36g

95. Shrimp Pineapple

Preparation Time: 15 minutes.
Cooking Time: 15 minutes.
Serving: 4
Ingredients:
1 cup pineapple, chopped
1 pound raw jumbo shrimp
1 ½ tablespoon arrowroot starch
2 tablespoons avocado oil
Sauce:
1 tablespoon ginger, minced
2/3 cup pineapple juice
1 tablespoon garlic, minced
3 tablespoon sriracha
1 tablespoon soy sauce
2 teaspoons arrowroot starch
1 tablespoon garlic, minced
1 tablespoon honey
1/3 cup bell pepper, diced
Garnish:
Fresh green onion
Sesame seeds
Fresh limen
Directions:
Mix all the sauce ingredients in a bowl and keep it aside.
Toss shrimp with arrowroot in a bowl and shake off the excess.
Set a skillet with olive oil over medium heat.
Stir in pineapple chunks and cook for 5 minutes.
Transfer to a plate and keep them aside.
Sauté shrimp with avocado oil in the same skillet for 8 minutes.
Stir in bell peppers then sauté for 1 minute.
Add prepared sauce and mix well.
Stir in pineapple juice and chunks.
Cook for 30 seconds, then serve warm.
Serving Suggestion: Serve these shrimps with boiled white rice.
Variation Tip: Add garlic salt to the seasoning for more taste.

Nutritional Information Per Serving: Calories: 251 | Fat: 17g |Sodium: 723mg | Carbs: 21g | Fiber: 2.5g | Sugar: 2g | Protein: 7.3g

96. Fish Green Curry

Preparation Time: 15 minutes.
Cooking Time: 13 minutes.
Serving: 4
Ingredients:
1 (15-ounce can) coconut milk
2 tablespoons green curry paste
1 (1-inch) nub fresh ginger, peeled and grated
2 tablespoons lime juice
2 tablespoons fish sauce
1 crown broccoli, chopped
2 cups green beans, chopped
1 zucchini squash, chopped
2 pounds white fish
Salt, to taste
Serving:
Coconut milk yogurt
Chives
Directions:
Add coconut milk, lime juice, fish sauce, ginger, and curry paste to a cooking pot, and cook to a boil.
Stir in green beans and broccoli, and cook for 3 minutes. Stir fish and zucchini; cover and cook for 10 minutes. Serve warm.
Serving Suggestion: Serve the fish curry with cauliflower rice.
Variation Tip: Add olives or sliced mushrooms to the fish.
Nutritional Information Per Serving: Calories: 246 | Fat: 15g |Sodium: 220mg | Carbs: 40.3g | Fiber: 2.4g | Sugar: 1.2g | Protein: 12.4g

97. Poached Mahi Courgettes

Preparation Time: 15 minutes.
Cooking Time: 31 minutes.
Serving: 4
Ingredients:
4 (4-ounces) boneless mahi courgettes fillets
¼ teaspoon salt
1 cup olive oil
1 pound asparagus, trimmed
3 tablespoons olive oil
1 yellow onion, chopped
¼ teaspoon black pepper
1 pinch red pepper flakes
10 green olives, pitted and chopped

1 small head garlic, minced
1 cup jarred roasted red peppers, chopped
2 tablespoons capers, drained, chopped
½ cup dry white wine
½ cup fresh basil, chopped
1 tablespoon fresh lemon juice
Lemon wedges for serving

Directions:
At 250°F, preheat your oven.
Rub the fish with salt and keep it aside.
Add oil and fish to a skillet and sear for 3 minutes per side.
Bake this for 15 minutes, then cover and keep it warm.
Sauté onions with black pepper, pepper flakes, and oil in a skillet for 4 minutes.
Stir in red pepper, capers, garlic, and olives, then cook for 2 minutes.
Add wine and cook the mixture for 3 minutes on a simmer.
Stir in asparagus tips and cook for 1 minute.
Add lemon juice, parsley, and basil, then over the fish.
Garnish with lemon wedges.
Serve warm.
Serving Suggestion: Serve the fish with cauliflower rice.
Variation Tip: Replace mahi courgettes with codfish if needed.
Nutritional Information Per Serving: Calories: 392 | Fat: 16g |Sodium: 466mg | Carbs: 3.9g | Fiber: 0.9g | Sugar: 0.6g | Protein: 48g

98. Shrimp Salad

Preparation Time: 15 minutes.
Cooking Time: 17 minutes.
Serving: 2
Ingredients:
2 tablespoons olive oil
1/3 cup red onion, chopped
3 cups broccoli slaw
3 cups broccoli florets
1/2 teaspoon salt
2 garlic cloves, minced
½ pound shrimp, peeled and deveined
1 teaspoon lime juice
Green onions, chopped, for garnish
Cilantro, chopped
Sriracha and red pepper flakes, for garnish
Sesame almond dressing:
2 tablespoons almond butter

2 tablespoons water
1 tablespoon sesame oil
1 tablespoon tamari
1 tablespoon maple syrup
1 teaspoon lime juice
1 teaspoon ginger, minced
1 clove minced garlic
1 teaspoon sriracha sauce
¼ teaspoon black pepper

Directions:
Mix all the sesame almond dressing in a bowl.
Sauté onion with oil in a skillet for 5 minutes.
Stir in broccoli slaw and florest then sauté for 7 minutes.
Add black pepper and salt, then transfer to a plate.
Add minced garlic, shrimp, lime juice, and more oil to the same skillet.
Sauté for 5 minutes, then transfer the shrimp to the broccoli.
Pour the sesame dressing on top and garnish it with cilantro and green onions.
Serve warm.
Serving Suggestion: Serve the shrimp salad with cauliflower rice risotto.
Variation Tip: Add paprika for more spice.
Nutritional Information Per Serving: Calories: 212 | Fat: 9g |Sodium: 353mg | Carbs: 8g | Fiber: 3g | Sugar: 4g | Protein: 25g

99. Braised Lamb Shanks

Preparation Time: 15 minutes.
Cooking Time: 2 hr. 30 minutes.
Serving: 4
Ingredients:
1 ½ pounds eggplant, peeled
4 (12-ounce) lamb shanks, trimmed
2 tablespoons ground sumac
1 ¼ teaspoons salt
½ teaspoon black pepper
2 tablespoons olive oil
1 green bell pepper, diced
1 small onion, diced
3 garlic cloves, minced
5 plum tomatoes, diced
1 cup water
½ cup parsley, chopped
Directions:
Rub the lamb shanks with black pepper, salt, and 1 tablespoon sumac.

Sear lamb with 1 tablespoon oil in a large Dutch oven for 5 minutes per side.

Transfer the lamb to a plate.

Add the remaining 1 tablespoon oil, onion, minced garlic cloves, bell pepper, and 1 tablespoon sumac.

Sauté for 5 minutes, then return the lamb to the pot.

Stir in tomatoes, water and eggplant, then cook on a simmer for 2 hours.

Cover Remove the lid and cook for 10 minutes until the gravy thickens.

Garnish with parsley and serve warm.

Serving Suggestion: Serve the shanks with sweet potato salad.

Variation Tip: Add chopped green onion to the topping.

Nutritional Information Per Serving: Calories: 425 | Fat: 15g |Sodium: 345mg | Carbs: 12.3g | Fiber: 1.4g | Sugar: 3g | Protein: 23.3g

100.   Lamb Cabbage Rolls

Preparation Time: 15 minutes.
Cooking Time: 1 hr. 10 minutes.
Serving: 8
Ingredients:
½ cup bulgur, cooked
1 large head Savoy cabbage
2 tablespoons olive oil
2 cups onion, chopped
1 cup leeks, chopped
¾ teaspoon salt
¾ teaspoon black pepper
½ teaspoon ground turmeric
¼ teaspoon ground ginger
¼ teaspoon ground allspice
1 pinch ground cinnamon
12 ounces ground lamb
½ cup parsley, chopped
2 teaspoons fresh mint, chopped
1 large egg, beaten
½ cup white wine
½ cup chicken broth
2 teaspoons lemon zest, grated
3 tablespoons lemon juice
Directions:
At 325°F, preheat your oven.
Boil cabbage leaves in 2 ½ cups water in a cooking pan and drain.
Sauté onion and leeks with oil in a skillet for 8 minutes.

Add cinnamon, allspice, ginger, turmeric, black pepper, and salt, then cook for 1 minute.

Transfer this mixture to a bowl and add bulgur.

Stir in lamb, parsley, mint, and egg, then mix well.

Spread the cabbage leaves o the working surface.

Divide the lamb filling at the center of each leaf.

Wrap the leaves around the filling and place the wrap in a baking dish.

Add lemon juice, lemon zest, broth, and wine around the cabbage rolls.

Cover the dish with a foil sheet and bake for 1 hour in the oven.

Serve warm.

Serving Suggestion: Serve the rolls with roasted asparagus.

Variation Tip: Add a drizzle of parmesan cheese on top.

Nutritional Information Per Serving: Calories: 391 | Fat: 5g |Sodium: 88mg | Carbs: 3g | Fiber: 0g | Sugar: 0g | Protein: 27g

101.   Pan-Seared Beef and Mushrooms

Preparation Time: 15 minutes.
Cooking Time: 17 minutes.
Servings: 4
Ingredients:
1 ½ lb. lean beef, cubed
1/2 tablespoons Dash Desperation Seasoning
Nonstick cooking spray
4 cups mushrooms, sliced
1 cup beef broth
1 ½ teaspoon Garlic Gusto Seasoning
Directions:
Mix beef with seasoning and sauté in a skillet with cooking spray for 7 minutes.

Add broth and rest of the ingredients and cook for 10 minutes with occasional stirring.

Serve warm.

Serving Suggestion: Serve the beef with sweet potato salad.

Variation Tip: Drizzle parmesan cheese on top before serving.

Nutritional Information Per Serving: Calories: 255 | Fat: 12g |Sodium: 66mg | Carbs: 13g | Fiber: 2g | Sugar: 4g | Protein: 22g

102.   Lamb Pea Curry

Preparation Time: 15 minutes.
Cooking Time: 22 minutes.
Serving: 2
Ingredients:
1 ¼ cups jasmine rice
Cooking spray oil
14 ounces lean lamb medallions
5 teaspoons Thai green curry paste
1 red onion, sliced
14 ounces can creamy coconut evaporated milk
2 teaspoons fish sauce
1 ½ cups frozen peas
14 ounces mix carrot sticks, snow peas, and broccoli florets
Directions:
Sear the lamb with half of the curry paste and oil in a cooking pan for 2 minutes per side.
Cover this lamb and bake for 7 minutes at 400°F.
Meanwhile, sauté onion with remaining oil and curry pastes in a skillet for 1 minute.
Stir in fish sauce and milk, then cook for 5 minutes.
Add vegetables and cook for 5 minutes.
Slice the lamb and serve with veggies.
Enjoy.
Serving Suggestion: Serve the curry with toasted bread slices.
Variation Tip: Add crumbled feta cheese on top.
Nutritional Information Per Serving: Calories: 325 | Fat: 16g |Sodium: 431mg | Carbs: 22g | Fiber: 1.2g | Sugar: 4g | Protein: 23g

103.   Green Lamb Curry

Preparation Time: 15 minutes.
Cooking Time: 2 hrs. 30 minutes.
Serving: 2
Ingredients:
2/3 pound lean lamb, trimmed and diced
2 ½ tablespoons curry powder
½ teaspoons salt
1 tablespoon vegetable oil
2 onions, sliced
4 garlic cloves, chopped
1 tablespoon tomato purée
½ pound fresh spinach
Small bunch coriander leaves, to serve
Black pepper, to taste
Directions:
Mix lamb meat with salt, black pepper, and curry powder in a bowl.

Sauté onions with oil in a skillet on medium heat until soft.
Stir in lamb and sauté until brown.
Add garlic, tomato puree and water then cover and cook for 2 hours on medium heat.
Remove the lid and cook for 20 minutes.
Stir in spinach and cook for 3 minutes.
Garnish and serve warm.
Serving Suggestion: Serve the curry with white rice.
Variation Tip: Add some kale leaves instead of the spinach
Nutritional Information Per Serving: Calories: 305 | Fat: 25g |Sodium: 532mg | Carbs: 2.3g | Fiber: 0.4g | Sugar: 2g | Protein: 18.3g

104.   Turkey Taco Soup

Preparation Time: 15 minutes.
Cooking Time: 45 minutes.
Serving: 6
Ingredients:
1 ½ pound lean ground turkey
1 onion, diced
1 (1 ¼ ounce) package taco seasoning
1 (1 ounce) package ranch dressing seasoning
1 (14oz) can chicken broth
1 (4 ounces) can diced green chiles
1 (15 ½ ounces) can whole kernel corn
1 (15 ½ ounces) can pinto beans
1 (15 ounces) can refried beans
1 (14 ½ ounces) can diced tomatoes with green chiles
1 (14 ½ ounces) can Mexican diced tomatoes

Directions:
Sauté onion and turkey in a skillet until golden brown.
Stir in the rest of the ingredients and cook for 45 minutes.
Serve warm.
Serving Suggestion: Serve the soup with toasted bread slices.
Variation Tip: Add zucchini noodles to the soup.
Nutritional Information Per Serving: Calories: 354 | Fat: 25g |Sodium: 412mg | Carbs: 22.3g | Fiber: 0.2g | Sugar: 1g | Protein: 28.3g

105.   Turkey Broccoli

Preparation Time: 15 minutes.
Cooking Time: 20 minutes.
Serving: 4
Ingredients:
1 tablespoon Dijon mustard

1 tablespoon whole grain mustard
1 cup chicken broth
4 teaspoons roasted garlic oil
4 cups broccoli florets
1 tablespoon garlic gusto seasoning
1½ pound boneless turkey breasts, diced
1 pinch dash desperation seasoning

Directions:
Mix broth with mustard in a bowl.
Sauté broccoli with oil and garlic gusto in a skillet for 2 minutes.
Transfer the broccoli to a bowl.
Sear the turkey bites in the same pan for 5 minutes per side.
Reduce heat, and stir in mustard mixture and broccoli.
Cover and cook for 7 minutes on a simmer.
Serve warm.
Serving Suggestion: Serve the chicken with a spinach salad.
Variation Tip: Add chopped green beans to the mixture.
Nutritional Information Per Serving: Calories: 388 | Fat: 8g |Sodium: 339mg | Carbs: 8g | Fiber: 1g | Sugar: 2g | Protein: 33g

106.   Sesame Chicken
Preparation Time: 15 minutes.
Cooking Time: 20 minutes.
Serving: 2
Ingredients:
1 pound boneless chicken breasts, diced
1 large head broccoli, chopped
2 red bell peppers, cut into chunks
1 cup snap peas
Salt and black pepper, to taste
Sesame seeds and green onions
Sauce:
¼ cup soy sauce
1 tablespoon sweet chili sauce
2 tablespoons honey
2 garlic cloves
1 teaspoon fresh ginger
Directions:
At 400°F, preheat your oven.
Mix all the sauce ingredients in a saucepan and cook until it thickens.
Remove the sauce from the heat and allow the sauce to cool.

Spread the veggies and chicken on a greased baking sheet.
Drizzle sauce over the mixture and mix well.
Bake the mixture for 20 minutes in the oven.
Garnish with sesame seeds.
Serve warm.
Serving Suggestion: Serve the chicken with toasted bread on the side.
Variation Tip: Add some canned corn to the meal.
Nutritional Information Per Serving: Calories: 334 | Fat: 16g |Sodium: 462mg | Carbs: 31g | Fiber: 0.4g | Sugar: 3g | Protein: 25.3g

107.   Spinach Mushroom Chicken
Preparation Time: 15 minutes.
Cooking Time: 43 minutes.
Serving: 4
Ingredients:
6 ounces bag raw spinach leaves
2 ounces cream cheese
2 garlic cloves, minced
8 ounces baby bella mushrooms
2 teaspoons garlic powder
2 teaspoons salt
2 teaspoons ground thyme
4 chicken breasts
4 mozzarella cheese slices
Directions:
At 400°F, preheat your oven.
Season chicken with thyme, salt, and 1 teaspoon garlic powder.
Place this chicken in a casserole dish and bake for 15 minutes in the oven.
Sauté garlic in a skillet for 1 minute.
Stir in spinach and cook for 10 minutes.
Add cream cheese, then mix well and remove from the heat.
Sauté mushrooms with thyme, salt, and 1 teaspoon garlic powder in a skillet for 7 minutes.
Stir in cream cheese mixture and mix well.
Spread this mixture on top of the baked chicken.
Drizzle cheese on top and bake for another 10 minutes.
Serve warm.
Serving Suggestion: Serve the chicken with toasted bread slices.

Variation Tip: Add butter sauce on top of the chicken before cooking.

Nutritional Information Per Serving: Calories: 419 | Fat: 13g | Sodium: 432mg | Carbs: 9.1g | Fiber: 3g | Sugar: 1g | Protein: 21g

108.   Grilled Buffalo Shrimp

Preparation Time: 15 minutes.
Cooking Time: 8 minutes.
Serving: 4
Ingredients:
11 ounces raw shrimp, peeled
1/4 cup Frank's Hot Sauce
1 tablespoon butter
Directions:
Mix butter with hot sauce in a bowl.
Thread the shrimp on the skewers and brush them with the butter mixture.
Grill these skewers for 2 minutes per side while basting with butter sauce.
Serve warm.
Serving Suggestion: Serve the shrimps with tomato ketchup.
Variation Tip: Coat the shrimp in breadcrumbs before cooking.
Nutritional Information Per Serving: Calories: 275 | Fat: 16g | Sodium: 255mg | Carbs: 1g | Fiber: 1.2g | Sugar: 5g | Protein: 19g

109.   Fire Cracker Shrimp

Preparation Time: 15 minutes.
Cooking Time: 6 minutes.
Serving: 4
Ingredients:
11 ounces raw shrimp, peeled
2 tablespoons Apricot Preserves
1 teaspoon lite soy sauce
½ teaspoon sriracha sauce
1 teaspoon sesame oil
Directions:
Place apricot in a small bowl and heat for 20 seconds in the microwave.
Mix oil, sriracha sauce, soy sauce, and apricot mixture in a bowl.
Thread the shrimp on the wooden skewers and brush them with apricot mixture.
Grill these skewers for 3 minutes per side.
Serve warm.
Serving Suggestion: Serve the shrimp with zucchini fries.

Variation Tip: Add crumbled cheese on top.
Nutritional Information Per Serving: Calories: 229 | Fat: 5g | Sodium: 510mg | Carbs: 37g | Fiber: 5g | Sugar: 4g | Protein: 21g

110.   Sheet Pan Chicken

Preparation Time: 15 minutes.
Cooking Time: 18 minutes.
Serving: 4
Ingredients:
1 ¾ pound boneless chicken breasts, diced
Salt, to taste
1 pound broccoli crowns
1 medium red bell pepper
2 tablespoons olive oil
¼ cup peanut butter
1 tablespoon tamari
1 tablespoon rice vinegar
1 tablespoon honey
juice from ½ lime
3 tablespoons water
1 pinch salt
Sesame seeds
Sliced green onions
Directions:
At 425°F, preheat your oven.
Layer 2 baking sheets with wax paper and grease with cooking spray.
Toss chicken, veggies, and all the ingredients in a large bowl.
Divide this mixture into the prepared baking sheet.
Bake the mixture for 18 minutes in the oven.
Garnish white sesame seeds and green onions.
Serve warm.
Serving Suggestion: Serve the chicken with a kale salad on the side.
Variation Tip: Coat the chicken with coconut shreds for a crispy texture.
Nutritional Information Per Serving: Calories: 384 | Fat: 15g | Sodium: 587mg | Carbs: 8g | Fiber: 1g | Sugar: 5g | Protein: 20g

111.   Chicken Thighs with Green Olive

Preparation Time: 15 minutes.
Cooking Time: 20 minutes. Serving: 4
Ingredients:
1 1/2 pound boneless chicken thighs, trimmed
¼ teaspoon salt - ¼ teaspoon black pepper
¼ cup all-purpose flour

3/4 cup cranberry juice
1 tablespoon olive oil
4 garlic cloves, minced
¾ cup chicken broth
1/4 cup dried cherries
¼ cup sliced green olives, pitted
2 tablespoons red-wine vinegar
1 tablespoon brown sugar
1 teaspoon dried oregano

Directions:
Rub the chicken with black pepper and salt, then coat with the flour.
Mix ¼ cup cranberry juice with 4 teaspoons flour in a bowl until smooth.
Sear the seasoned chicken in 1 tablespoon of oil in a skillet over medium heat for 5 minutes per side. Transfer the prepared chicken to a plate and keep it aside.
Stir in garlic and 1 teaspoon oil, and sauté for 30 seconds.
Add flour juice mixture, ½ cup cranberry juice, cherries, oregano, brown sugar, vinegar, and olives. Boil this mixture, reduce the heat, simmer, and cook for 6 minutes with occasional stirring.
Return this chicken to the pan and cook for 2 minutes. Serve warm.
Serving Suggestion: Serve the chicken with toasted bread slices.
Variation Tip: Add butter sauce on top of the chicken before cooking.
Nutritional Information Per Serving: Calories: 419 | Fat: 13g | Sodium: 432mg | Carbs: 9.1g | Fiber: 3g | Sugar: 1g | Protein: 33g

112. Chicken Divan

Preparation Time: 15 minutes.
Cooking Time: 41 minutes.
Serving: 8
Ingredients:
2 tablespoons olive oil
1 pound boneless chicken breast, diced
1 large onion, diced
3 garlic cloves, minced
¾ teaspoon salt
½ teaspoon black pepper
½ teaspoon dry thyme
¼ cup dry sherry
2 cups chicken broth
¼ cup all-purpose flour
2/3 cup Parmesan cheese, grated

¼ cup sour cream
2 pieces Broccoli crowns, chopped
½ cup water
3 tablespoons panko
½ teaspoon paprika

Directions:
At 400°F, preheat your oven.
Grease a 2 ½ quart baking dish with cooking spray.
Sauté chicken with 1 tablespoon of oil in a skillet until golden brown for 10 minutes.
Transfer to a plate, cover with a foil, and keep aside.
Sauté onion, thyme, black pepper, salt, and garlic with 2 teaspoons of oil in the same skillet for 4 minutes. Stir in sherry, then cook at a simmer for 3 minutes. Pour in 1 ½ cup broth then cook on a simmer with occasional stirring.
Mix flour with ½ cup broth in a bowl and pour into the skillet. Cook until the mixture thickens, then add sour cream and 1/3 cup parmesan. Return the chicken to the mixture and mix well Add broccoli and ½ cup water to a bowl, cover, and microwave for 2 minutes. Drain and transfer the broccoli to the chicken, then mix well. Spread this chicken mixture in the prepared casserole dish.
Drizzle remaining parmesan, panko, paprika, and 1 teaspoon of oil on top.
Bake for 22 minutes in the preheated oven.
Serve warm.
Serving Suggestion: Serve the chicken divan with roasted veggies on the side.
Variation Tip: Add peas and corn to the casserole.
Nutritional Information Per Serving: Calories: 334 | Fat: 16g | Sodium: 462mg | Carbs: 31g | Fiber: 0.4g | Sugar: 3g | Protein: 35.3g

113. Roasted Pork Chops

Preparation Time: 15 minutes.
Cooking Time: 16 minutes.
Serving: 6
Ingredients:
1 ½ teaspoons paprika
1 ½ teaspoon dried ginger
1 ½ teaspoon dried mustard
1 ½ teaspoon kosher salt
1 ½ teaspoon ground black pepper
1 ½ tablespoon olive oil
6 thick-cut bone-in pork chops
Ginger Green Beans:
1 ½ tablespoon olive oil
2 pounds green beans, de-stemmed

1/4 teaspoon crushed red pepper flakes

1 teaspoon dried ginger

3 teaspoons soy sauce

Directions:

At 500°F, preheat your oven.

Mix paprika, black pepper, brown sugar, kosher salt, dried mustard, and 1 teaspoon dried ginger in a bowl.

Rub the pork chops with the spice rub mixture.

Preheat a skillet with 1 tablespoon of oil over high heat.

Sear the pork chops for almost 2 minutes per side.

Roast these chops for 6 minutes in the oven and flip once cooked halfway through.

Meanwhile, sauté green beans with 1 tablespoon of olive oil in a skillet for 1 minute.

Stir in red pepper flakes, soy sauce and ½ teaspoons dried ginger, and cook for 5 minutes.

Serve the cooked pork chops with the green beans. Enjoy.

Serving Suggestion: Serve the pork chops with roasted green beans.

Variation Tip: Add paprika for more spice.

Nutritional Information Per Serving: Calories: 537 | Fat: 20g |Sodium: 719mg | Carbs: 25.1g | Fiber: 0.9g | Sugar: 1.4g | Protein: 37.8g

114.   Meatloaf

Preparation Time: 15 minutes.

Cooking Time: 9 minutes.

Serving: 6

Ingredients:

1 onion

1 ½ pound extra-lean ground beef

1 cup zucchini, shredded

¾ cup green pepper diced

1 egg

5 teaspoons Worcestershire sauce

3 teaspoons grainy mustard

2 tablespoons ketchup

½ cup breadcrumb

1 teaspoon smoked paprika

½ teaspoons salt

½ teaspoons black pepper

Directions:

At 375°F, preheat your oven.

Beat egg with black pepper, paprika, salt, Worcestershire sauce, and mustard in a large bowl.

Stir in breadcrumbs and vegetables.

Add beef, mix well and spread this meat mixture into a loaf pan.

Cover the meat mixture with ketchup on top.

Bake the meatloaf for 9 minutes in the oven.

Slice and serve warm.

Serving Suggestion: Serve the meatloaf with fresh green and mashed sweet potatoes.

Variation Tip: Skip zucchini and replace it with an equal amount of shredded carrot.

Nutritional Information Per Serving: Calories: 301 | Fat: 5g |Sodium: 340mg | Carbs: 24.7g | Fiber: 1.2g | Sugar: 1.3g | Protein: 15.3g

115.   Goan Fish Curry

Preparation Time: 15 minutes.

Cooking Time: 11 minutes.

Serving: 2

Ingredients:

3 garlic cloves, chopped

3 cm ginger, chopped

1 green chili, chopped

2 tomatoes, chopped

1 tablespoon coconut oil

1 red onion, diced

1 tablespoon garam masala

1 tablespoon ground cumin

1 x 400ml tin coconut milk

1 pound haddock fillet, cut into chunks

Juice 1 lime

½ bunch coriander, chopped

Directions:

Blend tomatoes with chili, ginger, and garlic in a food processor until smooth.

Sauté onion with oil in a wok for 2 minutes.

Stir in cumin and garam masala, then cook for 30 seconds.

Add the tomato mixture and coconut milk then boil the mixture.

Reduce the heat and cook for 2 minutes on a simmer.

Place the haddock pieces in the curry; cook for 6 minutes on a simmer.

Garnish with coriander and lime juice.

Serve warm.

Serving Suggestion: Serve the curry with cauliflower rice.

Variation Tip: Replace haddock with codfish if needed.

Nutritional Information Per Serving: Calories: 392 | Fat: 16g |Sodium: 466mg | Carbs: 3.9g | Fiber: 0.9g | Sugar: 0.6g | Protein: 48g

116. Salmon with Cherry Tomatoes

Preparation Time: 15 minutes.
Cooking Time: 31 minutes.
Serving: 4
Ingredients:
1 cup sweet onion, chopped
2 teaspoons garlic, minced
2 cups cherry tomatoes, halved
Salt and black pepper, to taste
1 ½ tablespoon balsamic vinegar
1 ½ tablespoon basil leaves, julienned
1 (2-lbs.) salmon fillet, cut into 4 pieces
Directions:
At 425°F, preheat your oven.
Sauté onion with 3 tablespoons olive oil in a sauté pan for 5 minutes.
Stir in garlic, then sauté for 1 minute.
Add ½ teaspoons black pepper, 1 teaspoon salt, and tomatoes, then cook for 15 minutes with occasional stirring.
Stir in basil and vinegar, then mix well.
Sear the salmon with olive oil in a skillet for 5 minutes per side.
Add the tomato mixture on top of the salmon.
Serve warm.
Serving Suggestion: Serve the salmon with fresh greens.
Variation Tip: Drizzle cheddar cheese on top for a rich taste.
Nutritional Information Per Serving: Calories: 351 | Fat: 4g |Sodium: 236mg | Carbs: 19.1g | Fiber: 0.3g | Sugar: 0.1g | Protein: 36g

117. Lemon White Fish Fillets

Preparation Time: 15 minutes.
Cooking Time: 10 minutes.
Serving: 2
Ingredients:
16 ounces cod fillets halibut
3 tablespoons olive oil
¼ teaspoon kosher salt
¼ teaspoon black pepper
2 lemons, cut in halves
Directions:
Rub the cod fillets with oil, black pepper, and salt, and place them in a skillet.
Cook this codfish for 2 minutes per side.
Drizzle lemon juice on top and cook for 3 minutes per side.

Enjoy.
Serving Suggestion: Serve the fish with roasted broccoli florets.
Variation Tip: Drizzle lemon zest on top before cooking.
Nutritional Information Per Serving: Calories: 415 | Fat: 15g |Sodium: 634mg | Carbs: 14.3g | Fiber: 1.4g | Sugar: 1g | Protein: 23.3g

118. Tuscan Chicken

Preparation Time: 15 minutes.
Cooking Time: 23 minutes.
Serving: 4
Ingredients:
1 pound boneless chicken breasts, sliced
2 tablespoons butter, spread
4 cups kale leaves, chopped
2 garlic cloves, chopped
1 package Knorr rice sides cheddar broccoli
¼ cup sun-dried tomatoes, sliced
Lemon wedges
Directions:
Rub the chicken with black pepper and salt.
Sear the chicken with 1 tablespoon butter in a skillet for 5 minutes per side.
Transfer this prepared chicken to a plate and keep it aside.
Sauté garlic and kale with remaining butter in the same skillet over medium-high heat for 3 minutes.
Stir in 2 cup water and cheddar broccoli, and tomatoes, then cook for 5 minutes with occasional stirring.
Return the cooked chicken to the skillet and cook for 5 minutes.
Garnish with lemon wedges and pine nuts.
Enjoy. Serving Suggestion: Serve the chicken with roasted veggies.
Variation Tip: Replace kale with baby spinach if needed.
Nutritional Information Per Serving: Calories: 369 | Fat: 14g |Sodium: 442mg | Carbs: 13.3g | Fiber: 0.4g | Sugar: 2g | Protein: 32.3g

119. Lean and Green Chicken Pesto Pasta

Preparation Time: 5 minutes
Cooking Time: 15 minutes
Servings: 1
Ingredients:
3 cups of raw kale leaves

2 tbsp. of olive oil
2 cups of fresh basil
1/4 teaspoon salt
3 tbsp. lemon juice
Three garlic cloves
2 cups of cooked chicken breast
1 cup of baby spinach
6 ounce of uncooked chicken pasta
3 ounces of diced fresh mozzarella
Basil leaves or red pepper flakes to garnish
Directions:
Start by making the pesto, add the kale, lemon juice, basil, garlic cloves, olive oil, and salt to a blender and blend until its smooth.
Add salt and pepper to taste.
Cook the pasta and strain off the water. Reserve 1/4 cup of the liquid.
Get a bowl and mix everything, the cooked pasta, pesto, diced chicken, spinach, mozzarella, and the reserved pasta liquid.
Sprinkle the mixture with additional chopped basil or red paper flakes (optional).
Now your salad is ready. You may serve it warm or chilled. Also, it can be taken as a salad mix-ins or as a side dish. Leftovers should be stored in the refrigerator inside an air-tight container for 3-5 days.
Nutrition: Calories: 244Protein: 20.5 gCarbohydrates: 22.5 gFats: 10 g

120.   Tomato Basil Salmon
Preparation Time: 10 minutes
Cooking Time: 20 minutes
Servings: 2
Total Time: 30 minutes
Ingredients:
2 tablespoons of grated Parmesan cheese
1 tablespoon of olive oil
1 tomato, should be thinly sliced
1 tablespoon of dried basil
2 (6 Ounce) of boneless salmon fillets
Directions:
Preheat your oven to 3750F (1900C). Get a baking sheet, line it with a piece of aluminum foil, and then spray with non-stick cooking spray. Put the salmon fillets in the foil and sprinkle with basil before you top it with tomato slices, drizzle olive oil over it, and then sprinkle again with Parmesan cheese (In that order).
Then put it in the already preheated oven and bake until the salmon becomes opaque at the center, and

the Parmesan cheese color changes to brown at the top — this should be around 20 minutes.
Nutrition: 405.4 Calories, 36.2g Protein, 4g Carbohydrate, 26.6 g Fat, Sodium: 179.5mg , Cholesterol: 103.5mg , Sugars: 1.7g

121.   Curry   Roasted Cauliflower
Preparation Time: 10 minutes
Cooking Time: 30 minutes
Servings: 4
Ingredients:
¼ cup of chopped cilantro to garnish
½ teaspoon of salt
½ teaspoon of cayenne
½ teaspoon of turmeric
1 teaspoon of garlic powder
2 teaspoon of curry powder
1 tablespoon of lemon juice
4 teaspoon of coconut oil, to be melted
6 cups of cauliflower florets
Directions:
Preheat your oven to 4500F
Get a resealable plastic bag or a large bowl and toss the cauliflower with salt, cayenne, turmeric, garlic powder, curry powder, lemon juice, and coconut oil.
Next is to get a foil-lined baking sheet and spread the cauliflower in a single layer. Roast, stir and flip over as frequently as possible until it becomes golden brown and tender in about 25-35 minutes.
Fill with fresh cilantro before serving.
Per Serving: 3 Green , 3 Condiments , 1 Healthy Fat

122.   Cauliflower   Rice Stuffing
Preparation Time: 10 minutes
Cooking Time: 15 minutes
Servings: 2
Ingredients:
½ teaspoon of salt
½ tablespoon of poultry seasoning
½ tablespoon of chopped fresh rosemary
1 tablespoon of chopped fresh sage
½ cup off chicken stock
4 cups of riced cauliflower
2 oz. of chopped walnuts
1/3 cup of diced yellow onion
1 cup of diced mushrooms
1 cup of diced celery
1 tablespoon of unsalted butter

Directions:

Get a large skillet and heat with medium heat. Add walnuts, onions, mushrooms, and celery; then sauté for about 5 minutes.

Add cauliflower rice and sauté for extra 2 minutes.

Next is to add seasoning and stock, then mix very well. Cover with the lid and let it cook until the liquid is absorbed in about 12-15 minutes.

Nutrition: 121 Calories, 24g Protein, 8g Carbohydrate, 6 g Fat

123.   Skinny Chicken Queso

Preparation Time: 10 minutes
Cooking Time: 15 minutes
Servings: 4
Ingredients:

2 ½ cups of celery sticks (13 oz.)

1, 1 lb. of bag mini sweet peppers, should be divided into 2 lengthwise with the stems and seeds removed.

½ cup of chopped cilantro (this is optional)

1 cup of diced tomatoes with green chilies

4 tablespoon of reduced-fat cream cheese

¾ cup of low-fat, plain Greek Yogurt

1 ½ cups of reduced-fat, shredded sharp cheddar cheese

12 oz. of shredded, cooked chicken breast

Directions:

Preheat your oven to 3500F

Remove the bell peppers and cilantro to one side, combine all of the remaining ingredients inside a bowl, and then pour inside a lightly greased casserole dish.

Let it bake for 20 minutes until it is thoroughly heated. Then serve hot with celery sticks and halved mini sweet peppers.

Per Serving: 3 Green , 1 Condiment , 1 Healthy Fat , 1 Leaner

Nutrition: 380 Calories, 45g Protein, 15g Carbohydrate, 15 g Fat

124.   Eggroll In A Bowl

Preparation Time: 5 minutes
Cooking Time: 5 minutes
Servings: 3
Ingredients:

½ cup of Green onions, needed to garnish

1 tablespoon of sesame oil

1/3 cup of soy sauce

1 teaspoon of ginger, should be minced

4 cloves of garlic, should be minced

12 ounces of shredded cabbage

1 ½ pound of ground turkey breast

Directions:

Get a bowl and combine soy sauce, ginger, and garlic and put aside. Put the turkey in a large skillet and apply medium heat to get it brown.

Next is to add the already shredded cabbage in it and stir very well to combine.

Then add the sauce mixture to the veggies and meat. Stir together and let it cook for about 3-5 minutes until the cabbage starts to wilt but remain crunchy

You can garnish with green onions if you like.

Nutrition: 231 Calories, 35g Protein, 12g Carbohydrate, 13 g Fat

125.   Chicken Cobb Salad

Preparation Time: 5 minutes
Cooking Time: 15 minutes
Servings: 2
Ingredients:

1 sachet of Optavia Puffed Ranch Snacks

Water to make it thin

1 teaspoon of dry ranch mix

¼ avocado, should be mashed

¼ cup of non-fat, plain Greek Yogurt

2 slices of cooked turkey bacon, should be chopped

1 cup of cherry tomatoes, should be halved

2 hard-boiled eggs, should be sliced

½ lb. of cooked chicken breast, should be cubed and sliced

4 cups of romaine or spring mix

Directions:

Get 2 salad bowls and divide the lettuce among them. Then, share the remaining salad toppings between the 2 salad bowls. To prepare the dressing, get a small bowl and combine water, ranch mix, avocado, and yogurt and mix very well to smooth.

Top the salads with Puffed Ranch Snacks and dressing and serve at once.

Nutrition: 125 Calories, 17g Protein, 9g Carbohydrate, 8 g Fat

126.   Roasted   Pork Tenderloin with Fresh Plum Sauce

Preparation Time: 10 minutes
Cooking Time: 50 minutes
Servings: 2
Ingredients:

1 teaspoon of cold butter

1 tablespoon of balsamic vinegar

1 cup of water

2 fruit (2-1/8" dia) firm plums, must be pitted and both cut into 4

3 sprig (blanks) of fresh thyme sprigs, or more if desired

2 eaches of shallots, should be sliced

1 red onion, should be sliced

1 tablespoon of vegetable oil

Ground pepper and salt to taste

1 pork tenderloin

Directions:

Preheat your oven to 400°F (200°C). You should thoroughly season the pork tenderloin with black pepper and salt

Put the oil in a large, oven-proof skillet and heat over medium-high heat. Then cook the tenderloin until it becomes brown on all sides, using about 2-4 minutes for each side. Next is to move the tenderloin to a small plate.

Sauté the sliced onion with a pinch of salt inside the same skillet till it becomes soft in about 3-5 minutes. You should add the shallots at this stage and reduce the heat from the oven to medium, stir while it continues to cook for about 10 minutes or until the onions and shallots become golden brown and caramelized. Stir the thyme inside the onion mixture, put the tenderloin on the onion mixture, skin-side down, and set plum quarters around the pork tenderloin. Transfer the skillet to the already preheated oven.

You will have to cook until the pork center becomes a little bit pink in about 20 minutes. At this stage, if you insert an instant-read thermometer at the center, its readings should be about 145°F (63°C). Then move the plums and pork inside a plate.

Now, put the skillet on medium-high heat and pour balsamic vinegar and water inside the mixture. Get the mixture to boil and scrape the browned side of the food with a spoon. Then, cook and stir until the liquid is reduced by 50% in about 5-10 minutes and remove from the heat. Add butter into the mixture till it becomes melted and the sauce starts to shine. Then pour the shiny sauce over the plums and porks.

Nutrition: 370.2 Calories, 37.4g Protein, 22.5g Carbohydrate, 14.5 g Fat, Sodium: 182.4mg , Cholesterol: 103.6mg , Sugars: 11.6g

127. Alaskan Cod and Shrimp with Fresh Tomato

Preparation Time: 10 minutes

Cooking Time: 15 minutes

Servings: 6

Ingredients:

1 tablespoon of dried oregano, or as needed

Salt to taste

½ pound of large shrimp, should be peeled and deveined

1 pound of Alaskan cod

1 teaspoon of dried oregano

5 large tomatoes, to be chopped

6 cloves of garlic, should be minced

2 tablespoons of olive oil

Directions:

Put the oil in a skillet and heat over medium-high heat, cook, and continue to stir the garlic inside the oil until it becomes golden brown, but avoid getting it burned. Next is to add the tomatoes and mix until their juices are released. Then add 1teaspoon of oregano while stirring.

Put the shrimp and cod on the tomato mixture and season it with salt. Put a lid over the skillet to cover and allow it to simmer for 3 minutes. Turn the cod to the other side and season with 1 tablespoon of oregano and salt, cover it again and cook for another 3 minutes. Remove the lid and cook it while opened till its juice evaporates in about 2-3 minutes.

Nutrition: 165.8 Calories, 21.3g Protein, 7.6g Carbohydrate, 5.7 g Fat, Sodium: 128.1mg , Cholesterol: 85.3mg , Sugars: 4.1g

128. Simple Lemon Herb Chicken

Preparation Time: 10 minutes

Cooking Time: 15 minutes

Servings: 2

Ingredients:

2 sprigs of fresh parsley, needed for garnishing

1 pinch of dried oregano

1 tablespoon of olive oil

Pepper and salt to taste

1 lemon

2 breast half, where the bone and skin must have been removed

Directions:

Cut the lemon into half, and squeeze juice from one of the halves on the chicken. Then season with salt to taste. Put your oil in a small skillet and apply medium-low heat

As soon as the oil becomes hot, put the chicken inside and as the chicken is being sautéed, add oregano, pepper to taste, and the juice from the other half of the lemon. Sauté each side until the juice gets dried off in about 5-10 minutes. Serve with parsley to garnish.

Nutrition: 211.9 Calories, 28.8g Protein, 7.9g Carbohydrate, 8.6 g Fat, Sodium: 94.2mg , Cholesterol: 68.4mg , Sugars: 0.3g

129. Grilled Rosemary Chicken Breasts

Preparation Time: 35 minutes
Cooking Time: 10 minutes, Additional Time: 5 minutes
Servings: 4
Ingredients:
4 eaches of boneless, skinless chicken breast halves
1/8 teaspoon of kosher salt
¼ teaspoon of ground black pepper
1 ½ tablespoon of lemon juice
1 ½ tablespoon of Dijon mustard
2 tablespoons of minced fresh rosemary
3 tablespoons of olive oil
8 cloves of garlic, should be minced
Directions:
Get an outdoor grill, oil the grate lightly, and preheat with medium-high heat.

Whisk salt, ground black pepper, lemon juice, mustard, rosemary, olive oil, and garlic together inside a large bowl.

Put the chicken breasts in a resealable plastic bag. Then pour the garlic mixture over the chicken; you should reserve about 1/8 of this mixture. Seal the bag and pour marinade over the chicken in a thorough manner. Then, leave it for about 30 minutes at room temperature.

Put the chicken in the already preheated grill and let cook for about 4 minutes. Flip the chicken and add the reserved marinade, do not stop grilling until it becomes thoroughly cooked in about 5 minutes. Cover it with foil and allow it to rest for 2 minutes before you serve.

Nutrition: 232 Calories, 26.7g Protein, 3.9g Carbohydrate, 11.6 g Fat, Sodium: 276mg , Cholesterol: 65.8mg , Sugars: 0.2g

130. Cauliflower with Kale Pesto

Preparation Time:5minutes
Cooking Time: 2 minutes
Servings: 6
Ingredients:
3 cups cauliflower, cut into florets
3 cups raw kale, stems removed
2 cups fresh basil
2 tablespoons extra virgin olive oil
3 tablespoons lemon juice
3 cloves of garlic
¼ teaspoon salt
Directions:
Put enough water in a pot and bring to a boil over medium flame. Blanch the cauliflower for 2 minutes. Drain then place in a bowl of ice-cold water for 5 minutes. Drain again.

In a blender, add the rest of the ingredients. Pulse until smooth.

Pour over the pesto over the cooked cauliflower.

Nutrition: Calories: 41; Protein: 1.8g; Carbs: 5g; Fat: 5.3g; Sugar: 1.4g

Chapter 4:

Soup

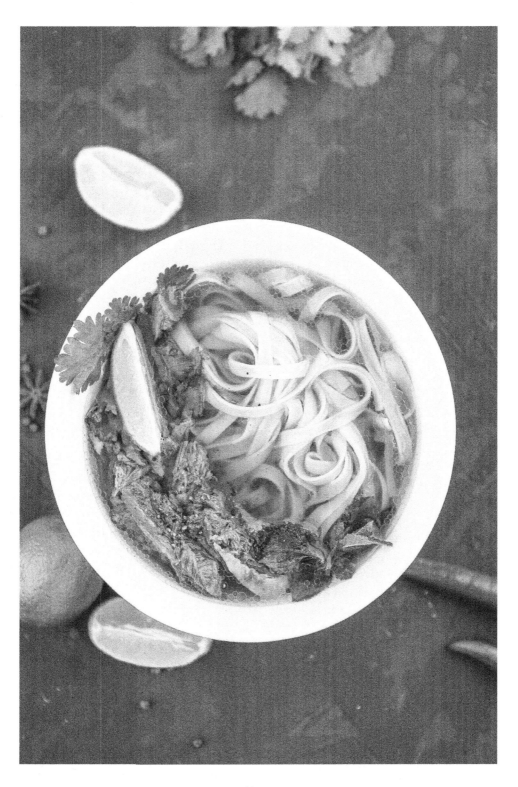

131. Instant Pot® Hamburger Soup

(Ready in 1 hour and 10 minutes, Serve 8, Difficulty: Normal)

Nutrition per Serving: Calories: 112, Protein: 18.7 g, Carbohydrates: 17.8 g, Fat: 11.2 g, Cholesterol: 51.7 mg, Sodium: 950.4 mg.

Ingredients:

680 g of ground beef 1 medium onion, finely chopped 3(14.5 ounces) cans of beef consommé 1(28 ounces) can of diced tomatoes 2 cups of water 1(10.75 ounces) can of condensed tomato soup 4 carrots, finely chopped 3 stalks of celery, finely chopped 4 tablespoons of pearl barley ½ teaspoon of dried thyme bay leaf

Instructions:

Switch on a multi-functional pressure cooker and select the cook mode (such as Instant Pot®). Cook and stir until browned, 5-10 minutes, with the beef and onion. Pour the beef, onions, water, and tomato soup into the mixture. Add some celery, onions, barley, thyme, and bay leaf. 2. Cover the lid and lock it. Pick "Feature Soup," set the timer to 30 minutes. Allow pressure to build for 10-15 minutes. 3. The release pressure is about 10 minutes using the natural-release method as instructed by the manufacturer.

132. Chef John's Butternut Bisque

(Ready in 50 minutes, Serve 6, Difficulty: Normal)

Nutrition per Serving: Calories: 213, Protein: 3.2 g, Carbohydrates: 27.1 g, Fat: 13.7 g, Cholesterol 45.8 mg, Sodium: 1058.9 mg.

Ingredients:

3 tablespoons of butter 1 large onion, diced 1 teaspoon of kosher salt, plus more to taste, divided 1(907 g) butternut squash 2 tablespoons of tomato paste quart of chicken broth 1 pinch of cayenne pepper tablespoons of maple syrup, or to taste ½ cup of heavy cream or crème fraiche Pomegranate seeds For Garnish: Some heavy cream or crème fraiche Chopped fresh chives.

Instructions:

Over medium-low pressure, melt butter in a pot. Put in the onions and a huge pinch of salt. Cook and stir until the onions, around 10-15 minutes, have softened but not taken on any color. 2. Cut off the squash ends. Carefully cut the squash lengthwise in ½ and remove the seeds. Using a potato peeler, peel the squash. Slice into chunks. 3. Raise the heat to medium-high below the pot. In the tomato paste, stir, simmer, and stir until the mixture starts to caramelize and brown for about 2 minutes. Add the potato, 1 teaspoon of salt, chicken broth, and cayenne pepper. Bring to a boil, reduce heat to medium-low, and simmer, 15-25 minutes, until the squash is very tender. Reduce heat to low levels. Blend until very creamy with an immersion blender. Add the cream and maple syrup and if needed, add more salt. 4. Ladle into bowls for serving. garnish with a cream swirl and a scattering of pomegranate seeds and chives.

133. California Italian Wedding Soup

(Ready in 25 minutes, Serve 6, Difficulty: Easy)

Nutrition per Serving: Calories: 159, Protein: 11.5 g, Carbohydrates: 15.4 g, Fat: 5.6 g, Cholesterol:55.3 mg, Sodium: 98.6 mg.

Ingredients:

226 g of extra-lean ground beef egg, lightly beaten tablespoons of Italian-seasoned breadcrumbs 1 tablespoon of grated parmesan cheese tablespoons of shredded fresh basil leaves 1 tablespoon of chopped Italian flat-leaf parsley (Optional) 2 green onions, sliced (Optional) 5 ¾ cups of chicken broth 2 cups of finely sliced escarole (spinach may be substituted) 1 lemon, zested ½ cup of orzo (rice-shaped pasta), uncooked For Topping: Grated parmesan cheese

Instructions:

The meat, egg, parsley, bread crumbs, cheese, basil, and green onions are mixed to form 3/4-inch balls. 2. Over high heat, pour the broth into a large saucepan. Drop into meatballs while boiling. Stir in escarole, orzo, and lemon zest. Return to a boil and reduce to medium heat. Cook for 10 minutes on a slow boil or until the orzo is tender, stirring frequently. Serve with cheese.

134. Thai Red Curry Chicken Soup

(Ready in 45 minutes, Serve 6, Difficulty: Normal)

Nutrition per Serving: Calories: 130, Protein: 16.4 g, Carbohydrates: 16.8 g, Fat: 23.1 g, Cholesterol: 36.8 mg, Sodium: 662.9 mg.

Ingredients:

2 tablespoons of red curry paste red bell pepper, thinly sliced 1 small onion, chopped 1(14 ounces) can

of coconut milk 1 tablespoon of fish sauce cups of homemade chicken stock cups of shredded cooked chicken 1 ½ cups of cooked basmati rice tablespoons of chopped fresh cilantro

Instructions:

Cook the curry paste over medium-high heat in a large, heavy saucepan until the oils are set to release, 1-2 minutes. Add the red pepper and onion and cook for about 5 minutes, stirring, until tender. Stir in coconut milk until mixed well. Add the fish sauce, and then the stock of chicken. 2. Lower the heat and simmer for 15 minutes. Add cooked rice and chicken. Stir over heat until thoroughly warmed. Right before serving, add chopped cilantro.

135.   Geneva's   Ultimate Hungarian Mushroom Soup

(Ready in 50 minutes, Serve 6, Difficulty: Normal)
Nutrition per Serving: Calories: 14, Protein: 7 g, Carbohydrates: 16.2 g, Fat: 7 g, Cholesterol: 18.9 mg, Sodium: 573.1 mg.

Ingredients: 2 tablespoons of unsalted butter 2 cups of chopped onions 680 g of fresh mushrooms, thickly sliced 4 ½ teaspoons of chopped fresh dill tablespoon of Hungarian sweet paprika 1 tablespoon of soy sauce cups of low-sodium chicken broth 1 cup of skim milk tablespoons of all-purpose flour ½ ripe tomato ½ Hungarian wax pepper teaspoon of salt Ground black pepper, to taste ½ cup of light sour cream.

Instructions: In a large pot over medium heat, melt the butter. In the butter, cook and stir the onions until fragrant, about 5 minutes. Add the mushrooms and continue to cook for about 5 more minutes until the mushrooms are tender. Mix the mushroom mixture with the dill, paprika, soy sauce, and chicken broth, reduce the heat to low, cover and simmer for 15 minutes. 2. In a small bowl, whisk the milk and the flour together. In the soup, stir the mixture. Add the Hungarian wax and tomato pepper. Return the cover to the pot and simmer, occasionally stirring, for another 15 minutes. With salt and pepper, season. 3. In the soup, combine the sour cream and continue to cook and stir until the soup has thickened, 5-10 more minutes. Remove the pepper and tomato from the Hungarian wax and discard them before serving the soup.

136.   Vegan Red Lentil Soup

(Ready in 55 minutes, Serve 4, Difficulty: Normal)
Nutrition per Serving: Calories: 130, Protein: 13 g, Carbohydrates: 34.2 g, Fat: 14.6 g, Cholesterol: 0 mg, Sodium: 80.9 mg.

Ingredients:

tablespoon of peanut oil 1 small onion, chopped 1 tablespoon of minced fresh ginger root 1 clove of garlic, chopped 1 pinch of fenugreek seeds 1 cup of dry red lentils 1 cup of butternut squash, peeled, seeded, and cubed ⅓ cup of finely chopped fresh cilantro cups of water ½ (14 ounces) of can coconut milk 2 tablespoons of tomato paste teaspoon of curry powder 1 pinch of cayenne pepper 1 pinch of ground nutmeg Salt and pepper, to taste

Instructions:

Heat the oil and cook the ginger, garlic, onion, and fenugreek in a large pot over medium heat until the onion is tender. 2. Mix in the pot with the lentils, squash, and cilantro. Add the water, coconut milk, and tomato paste and stir. Use curry powder, nutmeg, cayenne pepper, salt, and pepper to season. 3. Bring to a boil, reduce heat to low, and simmer for 30 minutes or until tender with lentils and squash.

137.   Ham and Split Pea Soup Recipe-A Great Soup

(Ready in 1 hour and 50 minutes, Serve 8, Difficulty: Hard)
Nutrition per Serving: Calories: 237, Protein: 25.1 g, Carbohydrates: 37 g, Fat: 14.4 g, Cholesterol: 39.8 mg, Sodium: 1186.7 mg.

Ingredients:

2 tablespoons of butter ½ onion, diced 2 ribs of celery, diced 3 cloves of garlic, sliced 453 g of diced ham bay leaf 453 g of dried split peas 1 quart of chicken stock 2 ½ cups of water Salt and ground black pepper, to taste

Instructions:

Place the butter over medium-low heat in a large soup pot. Add the cabbage, celery, and sliced garlic and stir. Slowly cook until the onions, 5-8 minutes, are translucent but not brown. 2. Mix the ham, bay leaf, and split peas together. Sprinkle with chicken stock and water. Stir to mix, and cook gently, about 1 hour and 15 minutes, until the peas are soft and the soup is thick. Occasionally stir. 3. To serve, season with salt and black pepper.

138.   Beef Noodle Soup

(Ready in 50 minutes, Serve 6, Difficulty: Normal)
Nutrition per Serving: Calories: 377, Protein: 25.5 g,
Carbohydrates: 24.8 g, Fat: 19.4 g 3, Cholesterol: 89.3
mg 3, Sodium: 1039.7 mg.

Ingredients:
453 g of cubed beef stew meat cup of chopped onion
1 cup of chopped celery ¼ cup of beef bouillon
granules ¼ teaspoon of dried parsley 1 pinch of
ground black pepper 1 cup of chopped carrots 5 ¾
cups of water 2 ½ cups of frozen egg noodles
Instructions:
Sauté the stew beef, onion, and celery in a large
saucepan over medium-high heat for 5 minutes or
until the meat is browned on all sides. 2. Add the
bouillon, parsley, carrots, ground black pepper, and
pasta with water and eggs. Bring it to a boil, bring it
to low heat, and cook for 30 minutes.

139.   Butternut Squash Soup

(Ready in 1 hour, Serve 6, Difficulty: Normal)
Nutrition per Serving: Calories: 230, Protein: 6.9 g,
Carbohydrates: 59.7 g, Fat: 6.8 g, Cholesterol: 20.9
mg, Sodium: 1151.4 mg

Ingredients:
2 tablespoons of butter small onion, chopped 1 stalk
of celery, chopped 1 medium carrot, chopped
medium potatoes, cubed 1 medium butternut squash,
peeled, seeded, and cubed 1(32 fluid ounces)
container of chicken stock Salt and freshly ground
black pepper, to taste

Instructions:
In a large pot, melt the butter and fry the onion,
potatoes, celery, carrot, and squash for 5 minutes, or
until lightly browned. To cover the vegetables, add
plenty of chicken stock. Bring it to a boil. Reduce the
flame, cover the pot, and simmer for 40 minutes or
until all the vegetables are tender. 2. In a blender,
pass the soup and blend until creamy. 3. To achieve
the desired consistency, return to the pot and blend
in any remaining stock. With salt and pepper, season.

140.   Copycat Panera® Broccoli Cheddar Soup

(Ready in 1 hour and 5 minutes, Serve 8, Difficulty:
Normal)
Nutrition per Serving: Calories: 230, Protein: 14.3 g,
Carbohydrates: 10.7 g, Fat: 23 g, Cholesterol: 70.5
mg, Sodium: 624 mg.

Ingredients:
tablespoon of butter ½ onion, chopped ¼ cup of
melted butter ¼ cup of flour cups of milk cups of
chicken stock 1 ½ cup of coarsely chopped broccoli
florets 1 cup of matchstick-cut carrots 1 stalk of
celery, thinly sliced 2 ½ cups of shredded sharp
cheddar cheese Salt and ground black pepper, to
taste
Instructions:
In a skillet over medium-high heat, melt one
tablespoon of butter. Cook the onion in hot butter
for around 5 minutes until it is translucent. Only put
aside. 2. In a large saucepan, stir together 1/4 cup of
melted butter and flour over medium-low heat,
simmer until the flour loses its granular structure,
and add 1 to 2 tablespoons of milk, if necessary, 3-4
minutes to keep the flour from burning. 3. Pour milk
into the flour mixture gradually by continuously
whisking. Stir the chicken stock into a mixture of
milk. Bring to a boil, cook for about 20 minutes until
the flour flavor is gone and the mixture thickens.
Add the broccoli, carrots, sautéed onion, and celery
and boil for about 20 minutes until the vegetables are
soft. 4. Stir in the vegetable mixture with the cheddar
cheese before the cheese melts. To taste, season with
salt and pepper.

141.   Slow Cooker Creamy Chicken and Dumplings

(Ready in 5 hours and 15 minutes, Serve 8, Difficulty:
Hard)
Nutrition per Serving: Calories: 238, Protein: 17.3 g,
Carbohydrates: 37.9 g, Fat: 18.3 g, Cholesterol: 37.6
mg, Sodium: 1294 mg.
Ingredients:
4 skinless, boneless chicken breast halves 2 (10.75
ounces) cans of condensed cream of mushroom
soup onion, minced tablespoons of butter
tablespoons of rosemary Ground black pepper, to
taste 1 cup of vegetable broth, or as needed 2(10
ounces) packages of refrigerated biscuit dough, torn
into pieces
Instructions:
In a slow cooker, mix the chicken, mushroom soup
cream, rosemary, onion, butter, and black pepper
and add enough vegetable broth to fully cover the
ingredients. 2. Cook for 4 ½-5 ½ hours, on high. 3.
On top of the chicken mixture, arrange torn biscuit
dough, continue cooking until the dough is cooked
through about 30 minutes more.

142. Slow Cooker Lentil and Ham Soup

(Ready in 11 hours and 20 minutes, Serve 6, Difficulty: Hard)
Nutrition per Serving: Calories: 322, Protein: 15.1 g, Carbohydrates: 26.3 g, Fat: 6.1 g, Cholesterol: 19.7 mg, Sodium: 1169.6 mg.
Ingredients:
cup of dried lentils 1 cup of chopped celery 1 cup of chopped carrots 1 cup of chopped onion cloves of garlic, minced 1 ½ cups of diced cooked ham ½ teaspoon of dried basil ¼ teaspoon of dried thyme ½ teaspoon of dried oregano 1 bay leaf ¼ teaspoon of black pepper 32 ounces of chicken broth 1 cup of water 8 teaspoons of tomato sauce
Instructions:
Mix the lentils, carrots, celery, cabbage, garlic, and ham in a three ½-quart or larger slow cooker. Using basil, thyme, oregano, bay leaf, and pepper to season. Stir in the chicken broth, tomato sauce, and water. 2. Cover and simmer for 11 hours on low pressure. Before serving, discard the bay leaf.

143. Avocado Soup with Chicken and Lime

(Ready in 30 minutes, Serve 6, Difficulty: Easy)
Nutrition per Serving: Calories: 129, Protein 16.5 g, Carbohydrates: 24.9 g, Fat: 15.3 g, Cholesterol: 37.3 mg, Sodium: 1047.6 mg.
Ingredients:
4(6 inches) of corn tortillas, julienned 1 ½ tablespoon of olive oil white onion, sliced thinly 8 cloves of garlic, thinly sliced 4 fresh jalapeno peppers, sliced 8 ounces of skinless, boneless chicken breast halves, cut into thin strips 1 quart of chicken broth ¼ cup of fresh lime juice 1 tomato, seeded and diced Salt and ground black pepper, to taste 1 avocado, peeled, pitted, and diced ¼ cup of chopped fresh cilantro
Instructions:
Preheat the oven to 400 degrees Fahrenheit (204 degrees Celsius). On a baking sheet, arrange the tortilla strips. 2. Bake in the preheated oven for 3-5 minutes, until finely browned. 3. Heat oil over low heat in a large saucepan. In oil, fry the onion, garlic, and jalapenos for 4-5 minutes until lightly browned. 4. Stir in the chicken, lime juice, chicken broth, onion, salt, and pepper. Simmer gently for about 10 minutes until the chicken is no longer pink. 5. Stir in the cilantro and avocado and heat for 3-5 minutes.

Change the seasonings according to taste. 6. Sprinkle with tortilla strips to serve. Ladle broth into cups.

144. Pho Ga Soup

(Ready in 30 minutes, Serve 6, Difficulty: Easy)
Nutrition per Serving: Calories: 162, Protein: 13.5 g, Carbohydrates: 32 g, Fat: 5.4 g, Cholesterol: 27.5 mg, Sodium: 148.9 mg.
Ingredients:
tablespoon of vegetable oil 1 small yellow onion, chopped 1(8 ounces) package of baby Bella mushrooms, chopped 4 cloves of garlic, minced 8 cups of water 1(6.75 ounces) package of rice stick noodles 8 teaspoons of chicken bouillon cooked chicken breasts, shredded green onions, chopped ⅓ cup of fresh cilantro, chopped 2 cups of bean sprouts 1 lime, sliced into wedges 1 dash of Sirach hot sauce, or to taste.
Instructions:
Heat the vegetable oil over medium-high heat in a large saucepan and cook the onion, mushrooms, and garlic until tender, 5-10 minutes. Add the onion mixture to the broth, rice noodles, and chicken bouillon and bring to a boil. Reduce heat to low levels. 2. In chili, combine grilled chicken, green onions, and cilantro and cook for another 5 minutes. 3. Top with bean sprouts, a squeeze of lime juice, and Sirach hot sauce and transfer soup to serving bowls.

145. Spanish Garlic Soup

(Ready in 35 minutes, Serve 6, Difficulty: Easy)
Nutrition per Serving: Calories: 118, Proteins: 2.4 g, Carbohydrates: 10.9 g, Fat: 7.9 g, Cholesterol: 1.1 mg, Sodium: 1053.2 mg.
Ingredients:
2 tablespoons of olive oil head garlic, peeled and lightly crushed 6 cups of chicken stock carrots, cut into matchsticks 1 red bell pepper, thinly sliced Salt and pepper, to taste
Instructions:
Heat oil over low heat in a large saucepan. Stir in the garlic and simmer for about 5 minutes, until lightly browned. Pour in 1 cup of chicken stock, cover, and allow to simmer for about 10 minutes until the garlic is soft. 2. Mash the garlic into a coarse paste with a fork. Pour in the remaining chicken stock, bring to a boil and increase the heat to medium-high. 3. Add the carrots and cook for 1 minute, then add the red pepper and cook until the vegetables are tender. 4. Before eating, season with salt and pepper to taste.

146. Absolutely Ultimate Potato Soup

(Ready in 50 minutes, Serve 8, Difficulty: Normal)
Nutrition per Serving: Calories: 129, Proteins: 12.6 g, Carbohydrates: 44 g, Fat: 41.5 g, Cholesterol: 91.2 mg, Sodium: 879.4 mg.

Ingredients:

453 g of bacon, chopped 2 stalks of celery, diced onion, chopped cloves of garlic, minced 8 potatoes, peeled and cubed cups of chicken stock, or enough to cover potatoes tablespoons of butter ¼ cup of all-purpose flour 1 cup of heavy cream 1 teaspoon of dried tarragon 3 teaspoons of chopped fresh cilantro Salt and pepper, to taste

Instructions:

Cook the bacon in a Dutch oven over medium heat until done. Take the bacon out of the grill, and set it aside. Drain the bacon fat from all but ¼ cup. 2. In the reserved bacon drippings, cook the celery and onion until the onion is translucent, about 5 minutes. Add the garlic, and proceed to cook for 1-2 minutes. To coat, add the cubed potatoes and toss. 3. Cook for between 3-4 minutes. Place the bacon back in the pan and add more chicken stock to cover the potatoes. Cover and boil until tender, then cook the potatoes. 4. Melt the butter over medium heat in a separate pan. Whisk the flour in. Cook for 1-2 minutes, continuously stirring. Heavy cream, tarragon, and cilantro are whisked in. Bring the cream mixture to a boil, and simmer until it thickens, stirring continuously. Into the potato mixture, stir the cream mixture. 5. Mash about 1/2 of the soup and return to the pan. Adjust the seasonings according to taste.

147. Healing Cabbage Soup

(Ready in 1 hour and 15 minutes, Serve 8, Difficulty: Normal)
Nutrition per Serving: Calories: 228, Proteins: 1.5 g, Carbohydrates: 8.6 g, Fat: 5.2 g, Cholesterol: 0 mg, Sodium: 435.9 mg.

Ingredients: 3 tablespoons of olive oil ½ onion, chopped 2 cloves of garlic, chopped 2 quarts of water 4 teaspoons of chicken bouillon granules teaspoon of salt, or to taste ½ teaspoon of black pepper, or to taste ½ head of cabbage, cored and coarsely chopped 1(14.5 ounces) can of Italian-style stewed tomatoes, drained and diced

Instructions: Heat olive oil over medium heat in a large stockpot. Stir in the onion and garlic and

simmer for about 5 minutes until the onion is clear. 2. Add sugar, bouillon, salt, and pepper and stir. Bring it to a boil, and add the cabbage. Simmer for about 10 minutes before the cabbage wilts. 3. Stir the tomatoes in. Return to the boil and simmer for 15-30 minutes, stirring regularly.

148. Chunky Chicken Noodle Soup

(Ready in 25 minutes, Serve 1, Difficulty: Easy)
Nutrition per Serving: Calories: 210, Proteins: 8.8 g, Carbohydrates: 13.2 g, Fat: 1.6 g, Cholesterol: 26.5 mg, Sodium: 1233.5 mg.

Ingredients:

3 quarts of water 1(32 fluid ounces) container of chicken stock 8 cubes of chicken bouillon 3 skinless, boneless chicken breast halves, cut into 1-inch pieces 4 cups of egg noodles cup of frozen peas and carrots carrots, chopped stalks of celery, chopped ¼ cup of chopped onion 1 teaspoon of salt 1 teaspoon of ground black pepper ¼ teaspoon of dried basil ⅛ teaspoon of crushed bay leaf ⅛ teaspoon of dried oregano

Instructions:

In a large stockpot, put the water, chicken stock, and chicken bouillon to a boil. Put in the chicken breast, the egg noodles, the peas and vegetables, the sliced carrots, the celery, the onion, the garlic, the black pepper, the basil, the bay leaves, and the oregano. 2. Continue to simmer for 20 minutes, uncovered. Reduce the heat to mild and cook until the chicken in the center is no longer pink and the noodles are soft, 5-10 more minutes.

149. Thai Chicken Cabbage Soup

(Ready in 45 minutes, Serve 6, Difficulty: Normal)
Nutrition per Serving: Calories: 227, Proteins: 20.8 g, Carbohydrates: 42.3 g, Fat: 3.1 g Cholesterol: 61.3 mg, Sodium: 118.3 mg.

Ingredients:

3 skinless, boneless chicken breast halves 8 cups of chicken broth 2 leeks, sliced 6 carrots, cut into 1-inch pieces medium head cabbage, shredded 1(8 ounces) package of uncooked egg noodles 1 teaspoon of Thai Chile sauce

Instructions:

Place the chicken breasts in a stockpot or Dutch oven with the broth. Bring to a boil and simmer for 20 minutes or until the chicken is fully cooked. To cool, remove the chicken from the broth and set it aside. 2. In the pot, place the leeks and carrots and simmer for 10 minutes, or until tender. Into bite-sized bits, shred the cooled chicken and return it to the pot. 3. Add the noodles to the cabbage and egg and simmer for another 5 minutes or until the noodles are tender. Like a stew, the broth should be thick. 4. Serve hot with Thai chili sauce and season to taste

150.   Portuguese Chicken Soup II

(Ready in 40 minutes, Serve 6, Difficulty: Normal)
Nutrition per Serving: Calories: 159, Proteins: 16.8 g, Carbohydrates: 6.8 g, Fat: 7.1 g, Cholesterol: 49.1 mg, Sodium: 63.2 mg.

Ingredients:

whole bone-in chicken breast, with skin 1 onion, cut into thin wedges 4 sprigs fresh parsley ½ teaspoon of lemon zest 1 sprig fresh mint 6 cups of chicken stock ⅓ cup of thin egg noodles tablespoons of chopped fresh mint leaves Salt, to taste ¼ teaspoon of freshly ground white pepper

Instructions:

Simmer the chicken breast in stock in a large saucepan with the onion, lemon zest, parsley, and mint sprig until cooked, about 35 minutes. 2. Cool, remove the breast, then peel the meat off and cut it into julienne. 3. Strain the broth, bring it back to the pot, and bring it to a boil. Pasta and chopped mint are included. Season with salt and white pepper to taste. Heat before the al dente pasta is cooked. 4. Stir in the lemon juice and chicken julienne, and remove from the heat. Ladle it into soup dishes and cover it with lemon and mint leaf pieces.

151.   Creamy Italian White Bean Soup

(Ready in 50 minutes, Serve 4, Difficulty: Normal)
Nutrition per Serving: Calories: 124, Proteins: 12 g, Carbohydrates: 38.1 g, Fat: 4.9 g, Cholesterol: 2.4 mg, Sodium: 1014.4 mg.

Ingredients:

tablespoon of vegetable oil 1 onion, chopped 1 stalk of celery, chopped 1 clove of garlic, minced 2(16 ounces) cans of white kidney beans, rinsed and drained 1(14 ounces) can of chicken broth ¼ teaspoon of ground black pepper ⅛ teaspoon of dried thyme cups of water 1 bunch of fresh spinach, rinsed and thinly sliced 1 tablespoon of lemon juice.

Instructions:

Heat the oil in a large saucepan. In olive oil, fry the onion and celery for 5-8 minutes or until tender. Add the garlic and fry, constantly stirring, for 30 seconds. Add the rice, chicken broth, pepper, thyme, and 2 cups of water and blend well. Bring to a boil, reduce the heat and cook for 15 minutes, then simmer. 2. Remove 2 cups of the bean and vegetable mixture from the soup with a slotted spoon and set it aside. 3. Combine remaining soup in small batches in the blender at low speed until smooth (it helps remove the centerpiece of the blender cover to allow steam to escape.) Until blended, pour soup back into the stockpot and mix in the reserved beans. 4. Bring it to a boil, stirring regularly. Add the spinach and simmer for 1 minute or until the spinach wilts. Remove from heat and serve on top of fresh grated parmesan cheese. Stir in lemon juice.

152.   Southwestern Turkey Soup

(Ready in 45 minutes, Serve 8, Difficulty: Normal)
Nutrition per Serving: Calories: 218, Proteins: 13.5 g, Carbohydrates: 11.9 g, Fat: 9.8 g, Cholesterol: 32.5 mg, Sodium: 632 mg.

Ingredients:
½ cups of shredded cooked turkey 4 cups of vegetable broth 1(28 ounces) can of whole peeled tomatoes 1(4 ounces) can of chopped green Chile peppers 2 Roman (plum) tomatoes, chopped onion, chopped cloves of garlic, crushed 1 tablespoon of lime juice ½ teaspoon of cayenne pepper ½ teaspoon of ground cumin Salt and pepper, to taste 1 avocado, peeled, pitted, and diced ½ teaspoon of dried cilantro 1 cup of shredded Monterey Jack cheese.

Instructions:

Combine the turkey, broth, dried tomatoes, fresh tomatoes, green chilies, ginger, garlic, and lime juice in a large pot over medium heat. Use cayenne, cinnamon, and pepper to season. Bring it to a boil, reduce the flame, and simmer for 15 to 20 minutes. 2. Add the cilantro and avocado and boil for 15 to 20 minutes, until lightly thickened. Spoon into bowls for cooking, then finish with melted cheese.

153.   Chicken Tortilla Soup I

(Ready in 40 minutes, Serve 8, Difficulty: Normal)
Nutrition per Serving: Calories: 377, Proteins: 23.1 g, Carbohydrates: 30.9 g, Fat: 19.1 g, Cholesterol: 46.1 mg, Sodium: 943.2 mg.

Ingredients: onion, chopped cloves of garlic, minced 1 tablespoon of olive oil teaspoons of chili powder 1 teaspoon of dried oregano 1(28 ounces) can of crushed tomatoes 1(10.5 ounces) can of condensed chicken broth 1 ¼ cup of water 1 cup of whole corn kernels, cooked 1 cup of white hominy 1(4 ounces) can of chopped green Chile peppers 1(15 ounces) can of black beans, rinsed and drained ¼ cup of chopped fresh cilantro 2 boneless chicken breast halves, cooked and cut into bite-sized pieces Crushed tortilla chips 1 avocado, sliced Shredded Monterey jack cheese Green onions, chopped

Instructions: Heat oil over low heat in a medium-sized stockpot. Cook the garlic and onion in the oil until tender. 2. Stir in the chili powder, onions, oregano, broth, and water. Bring it to a boil and let it simmer for 5-10 minutes. 3. Stir in the corn, chilies, beans, chicken, and cilantro. Simmer for 10 minutes . 4. Cover with crushed tortilla chips, avocado strips, cheese, and sliced green onion. Ladle soup into separate serving cups.

154.   Cheeseburger Soup I

(Ready in 50 minutes, Serve 8, Difficulty: Normal)
Nutrition per Serving: Calories: 121, Proteins: 18.9 g, Carbohydrates: 18.6 g, Fat: 18.3 g, Cholesterol: 80.9 mg, Sodium: 595.6 mg.

Ingredients:

226 g of ground beef ¾ cup of chopped onion ¾ cup of shredded carrots ¾ cup of chopped celery teaspoon of dried basil 1 teaspoon of dried parsley 4 tablespoons of butter cups of chicken broth cups of cubed potatoes ¼ cup of all-purpose flour 2 cups of cubed Cheddar cheese 1 ½ cup of milk ¼ cup of sour cream

Instructions:

In a large pot, melt one tablespoon butter or margarine over medium heat: cook and stir vegetables and beef until beef is brown. 2. Stir in basil and parsley. Add broth and potatoes. Bring to a boil, then simmer until potatoes are tender, about 10-12 minutes. 3. Melt the remainder of butter and stir in flour. Add the milk, stirring until smooth. 4. Gradually add milk mixture to the soup, stirring constantly. Bring to a boil and reduce heat to simmer. Stir in cheese. 5. When cheese is melted, add sour cream and heat through. Do not boil.

155.   Six Can Chicken Tortilla Soup

(Ready in 20 minutes, Serve 6, Difficulty: Easy)

Nutrition per Serving: Calories: 221, Proteins: 17.2 g, Carbohydrates: 27.2 g, Fat: 4 g, Cholesterol: 32 mg, Sodium: 1482.5 mg.

Ingredients:

1(15 ounces) can of whole kernel corn, drained 2(14.5 ounces) cans of chicken broth 1(10 ounces) can of chunk chicken 1(15 ounces) can of black beans 1(10 ounces) can of diced tomatoes with green Chile peppers, drained

Instructions:

Open the cans of rice, chicken broth, black beans, chunk chicken, green chilies, and sliced tomatoes. 2. In a big saucepan or stockpot, pour everything. Simmer until chicken is cooked over medium heat.

156.   Lentil and Buckwheat Soup

(Ready in 1 hour and 55 minutes, Serve 6, Difficulty: Normal)
Nutrition per Serving: Calories: 122, Proteins: 7.2 g, Carbohydrates: 28.9 g, Fat: 10 g, Cholesterol: 0 mg, Sodium: 191.7 mg.

Ingredients:

cup of brown lentils 1 tablespoon of olive oil 1 small onion, grated 1 small carrot, grated bay leaves 4 ½ cups of low-sodium vegetable broth, divided ¾ cup of raw buckwheat groats 1(9 ounces) package of fresh baby spinach tablespoons of extra-virgin olive oil

Instructions:

Soak the lentils for 1 hour in a bowl of cold water. Drain and set aside. 2. Heat oil over medium heat in a Dutch oven or heavy-bottomed stew pot. 3. Add the grated onion and carrot and sauté for 3 to 5 minutes, until tender. Add the lentils and bay leaves and mix until they are oil-coated. Pour 3 cups of vegetable broth into the mixture, stir and bring to a boil. Leave it for 10 minutes at a slow boil. 4. To a boil, reduce heat and add buckwheat. Simmer until soft but not mushy lentils and buckwheat is cooked over 25 minutes, if necessary, adding remaining broth. Remove from the heat and fold until wilted with fresh spinach. Remove the bay leaves. 5. Serve hot on top of each part with a 1/2 tablespoon of olive oil.

157.   Italian Wedding Soup I

(Ready in 50 minutes, Serve 6, Difficulty: Normal)
Nutrition per Serving: Calories: 216, Proteins: 27.3 g, Carbohydrates: 13.3 g, Fat: 14.2 g, Cholesterol: 86.8 mg, Sodium: 1211 mg.

Ingredients:

226 g of extra-lean ground beef egg, lightly beaten tablespoons of dry bread crumbs 1 tablespoon of grated Parmesan cheese ½ teaspoon of dried basil ½ teaspoon of onion powder 5 ¾ cups of chicken broth cups of thinly sliced escarole 1 cup of uncooked orzo pasta ⅓ cup of finely chopped carrot Instructions: Combine the beef, bacon, bread crumbs, cheese, and the basil and onion powder in a medium bowl. 2. Shape into 3/4-inch balls. 3. Heat the boiling broth in a large saucepan, stir in the escarole, orzo pasta, diced carrot, and meatballs. Return to boil, then reduce heat to medium. Cook for 10 minutes at a slow boil, or until the pasta is al dente. To prevent sticking, stir frequently.

158. Cheese Soup with Broccoli

(Ready in 1 hour and 5 minutes, Serve 7, Difficulty: Normal)

Nutrition per Serving: Calories: 349, Proteins: 20.8 g, Carbohydrates: 22.8 g, Fat: 19.5 g, Cholesterol: 38.4 mg, Sodium: 1538.3 mg.

Ingredients:

onion, chopped 6 tablespoons of margarine ⅓ cup of all-purpose flour Salt and pepper, to taste 4 cups of milk cups of chicken broth 1 carrot, shredded 1 cup of broccoli florets ½ cup of chopped celery 453 g of processed cheese food (e.g., Velveeta®), cubed Instructions:

Cook the onions in the butter or margarine until tender in a large saucepan over medium-high heat. Stir in the flour, salt, and pepper to taste. 2. Until smooth, blend. Slowly add the cream until the mixture is thick and bubbling. 3. Bring the chicken broth to a boil in a smaller saucepan. Add the carrot, broccoli, and celery. Cook for approximately 5 minutes, or until tender. Combine the mixture of the broth with the mixture of the milk and whisk until thoroughly mixed. 4. Put some cheese. Allow the soup to heat until the cheese is melted over medium heat. Important: Do not let the soup boil because the soup becomes separated and curdled by the cheese. Serve warm and enjoy it!

159. Brussels Sprouts Soup with Caramelized Onions

(Ready in 1 hour and 10 minutes, Serve 4, Difficulty: Normal)

Nutrition per Serving: Calories: 112, Proteins: 7.2 g, Carbohydrates: 31.5 g, Fat: 10.5 g, Cholesterol: 13.4 mg, Sodium: 801.3 mg.

Ingredients:

tablespoon of olive oil onions, thinly sliced 1 tablespoon of sugar 453 g of Brussels sprouts, trimmed and halved 1 teaspoon of fresh thyme cups of chicken stock Salt and ground black pepper, to taste ½ cup of sour cream dashes hot pepper sauce (such as Frank's Red-Hot®), or to taste Instructions: Combine the oil and onions over low heat in a pot. Cover and cook for 30-40 minutes, until very tender and smooth. Remove the cover and sprinkle the onions with sugar. Cook, uncovered, 10-15 minutes longer until the onions are light brown. 2. Stir the Brussels sprouts and thyme into the pot. Pour in the stock and add salt and pepper to the soup for seasoning. Bring to a boil, reduce the heat, and cook for around 10 minutes until the sprouts are just tender. 3. Allow the broth to cool. Blend with an immersion blender to a perfect consistency. 4. Reheat gently for about 2 minutes and if necessary, adjust the seasoning. 5. Using a spoonful of sour cream and a hot pepper sauce dash to finish the soup.

160. Potato-Parsnip Soup with Crème Fraiche and Bacon

(Ready in 1 hour and 35 minutes, Serve 6, Difficulty: Hard)

Nutrition per Serving: Calories: 277, Proteins: 7.8 g, Carbohydrates: 46.4 g Fat: 30.9 g, Cholesterol: 81.7 mg, Sodium: 617.8 mg.

Ingredients:

680 g of potatoes, peeled and cut into chunks 453 g of parsnips, peeled and cut into chunks onion, cut into large chunks cloves of garlic, quartered tablespoons of extra-virgin olive oil 1 teaspoon of smoked paprika 1 teaspoon of salt Freshly ground black pepper, to taste 1(32 ounces) of carton low-sodium vegetable broth 1 pint of half-and-half 1 pinch of salt, to taste For Garnish: 1(7 ounces) of container crème Fraiche slices of bacon strips, cooked and crumbled ¼ cup of chopped fresh chives Instructions:

The oven should be preheated to 425 degrees Fahrenheit (218 degrees Celsius). With parchment paper, cover a rimmed baking sheet. 2. On the prepared baking sheet, spread the potatoes, parsnips, onions, and garlic cloves drizzle the top with olive oil. Use paprika, salt, and pepper to season. Toss until evenly coated and spread back out into an even layer. 3. Roast in the preheated oven for about 40 minutes, until browned in spots. 4. Place the roasted vegetables in a large pot. Cover with vegetable broth. Cook until the vegetables are very tender, about 30 minutes. Bring to a simmer. Remove from the heat. 5. Use an immersion blender to gently blend the hot soup until smooth. Stir in half-and-a-half when well-integrated. Season with salt. 6. Soup with a ladle into bowls. With dollops of crème Fraiche, bacon bits, and chives, garnish each bowl.

161. Creamy Chicken and Wild Rice Soup

(Ready in 25 minutes, Serve 8, Difficulty: Easy)
Nutrition per Serving: Calories: 236, Proteins: 12 g, Carbohydrates: 22.6 g, Fat: 36.5 g, Cholesterol: 135.1 mg, Sodium: 996.9 mg.

Ingredients:
4 cups of chicken broth 2 cups of water 2 cooked, boneless chicken breast halves, shredded 1(4.5 ounces) package of quick-cooking long grain and wild rice with seasoning packet ½ teaspoon of salt ½ teaspoon of ground black pepper ¾ cup of all-purpose flour ½ cup of butter 2 cups of heavy cream Instructions:
Combine the broth, water, and chicken in a large pot over medium heat. Only bring it to a boil, then stir in the rice and reserve the seasoning packet. Cover and Remove from the heat. 2. Combine the salt, pepper, and flour in a small bowl. Melt the butter in a medium saucepan over medium heat. Stir in the contents of the packet of seasoning until the mixture is bubbly. 3. Reduce the heat to low, then whisk in the tablespoons of the flour mixture to form a roux. Whisk in the cream, a little at a time, until smooth and fully incorporated. Cook for 5 minutes until it thickens. 4. Stir the mixture of milk into the broth and rice. Cook for 10-15 minutes over medium heat until thoroughly cooked.

162. Joe's Homemade Mushroom Soup

(Ready in 20 minutes, Serve 20, Difficulty: Easy)
Nutrition per Serving: Calories: 227, Proteins: 8.7 g, Carbohydrates: 16.5 g, Fat: 15 g, Cholesterol: 41.5 mg, Sodium: 314.8 mg.

Ingredients:
¼ cup of butter large onion, chopped 2268 g of sliced fresh mushrooms 1 ¼ cup of all-purpose flour

2 ½ teaspoons of ground black pepper 1 ½ teaspoon of salt 10 cups of milk 10 cups of chicken broth ½ cup of minced fresh parsley 1 pinch ground nutmeg, or to taste ¼ cup of sour cream, oras needed Instructions:
Over medium heat, melt the butter in a large saucepan. In hot butter, cook and stir the onion and mushroom for about 3 minutes until the onion is tender. Stir in the onion mixture with flour, pepper, and salt. 2. Stream milk and chicken broth into the mixture steadily when stirring. 3. Bring the liquid to a boil and simmer for about 2 minutes, until it thickens. Remove the saucepan from the heat. Stir in the broth with parsley and nutmeg. Bowls of ladle soup and top each with a dollop of sour cream.

163. Amazing Gnocchi Soup

(Ready in 30 minutes, Serve 6, Difficulty: Easy)
Nutrition per Serving: Calories: 127, Proteins: 18.1 g, Carbohydrates: 33.2 g, Fat: 9.4 g, Cholesterol: 42.4 mg, Sodium: 490.6 mg.

Ingredients:
cups of water 1 ¼ cups of potato gnocchi cooked chicken breast, chopped 1 small tomato, diced ⅓ onion, diced ½ cup of corn 1 green onion, chopped teaspoons of chicken bouillon granules broccoli stalks ¼ teaspoon of dried thyme ⅛ teaspoon of ground black pepper ⅛ teaspoon of salt 1 pinch of dried basil
Instructions:
Bring to a boil, combine water, gnocchi, ham, tomato, cabbage, maize, green onion, pepper, salt, chicken bouillon, broccoli, thyme, and basil. 2. Reduce heat and boil for about 15 minutes until gnocchi is cooked through and flavors are blended.

164. Cajun Scallop Chowder

(Ready in 30 minutes, Serve 4, Difficulty: Easy)
Nutrition per Serving: Calories: 235, Proteins: 37.1 g, Carbohydrates: 32.7 g, Fat: 9.5 g, Cholesterol: 91.1 mg, Sodium: 1398.1 mg.

Ingredients:
1(16 ounces) package mixed frozen vegetables (broccoli, corn, red pepper) 2 tablespoons of butter ¾ cup of chopped onion clove of garlic, minced 1(4 ounces) package of sliced fresh mushrooms 1 tablespoon of Cajun seasoning tablespoons of all-purpose flour 1 ½ cups of milk 453 g of scallops, rinsed, drained, and cut in ½ 1 teaspoon of salt ⅛ teaspoon of ground black pepper

Instructions:

Place in a pot with enough water to cover the mixed vegetables and bring to a boil until the vegetables are tender around 5 minutes. Drain and set aside. 2. Over medium-low heat, melt the butter in a pot, cook and stir in the melted butter the onion, garlic, mushrooms, and Cajun seasoning until the onion is tender but not yet browned, around 5 minutes. Stir the flour in. 3. Pour in the milk, boil, and stir until the mixture thickens and begins to bubble. Add the scallops, salt, and pepper and continue to cook for 5-7 minutes until the scallops are opaque. Fold the vegetables into the mixture and simmer for-3 minutes before the vegetables are reheated. Immediately serve.

165.   Simple and Delicious Kale Soup

(Ready in 30 minutes, Serve 6, Difficulty: Easy)
Nutrition per Serving: Calories: 288, Proteins: 14.7 g, Carbohydrates: 43.9 g, Fat: 7.5 g, Cholesterol: 20.3 mg, Sodium: 1054.3 mg.

Ingredients:

tablespoon of butter 1 small onion, chopped cups of chicken broth 1 small tomato, chopped cups of loosely packed chopped kale 1 cup of canned white beans, rinsed and drained

Instructions:

Over medium-high heat, melt butter in a pot. Cook the onion in hot butter for 5-10 minutes, until soft. Stir in the onion with the chicken broth and tomato. 2. To near-boil, heat broth mixture and stir kale into liquid before fully submerged. Cook for 3-5 minutes before the kale wilts. 3. Stir the beans into the soup and simmer for another 2-3 minutes, until heated.

166.   Hearty Italian Meatball Soup

(Ready in 30 minutes, Serve 8, Difficulty: Easy)
Nutrition per Serving: Calories: 127, Proteins: 16.7 g, Carbohydrates: 30.8 g, Fat: 8.9 g, Cholesterol: 49.3 mg, Sodium: 498.1 mg.

Ingredients:

cups of water 2(14 ounces) cans diced tomatoes with onion and garlic, undrained 2(14 ounces) cans of beef broth teaspoon of Italian seasoning 1(16 ounces) package of frozen cooked Italian-style meatballs cups of frozen Italian-blend vegetables 1 cup of small star-shaped dried pasta ¼ cup of grated parmesan cheese

Instructions:

Stir together the water, onions, beef broth, and Italian seasoning in a large pot and bring to a boil. Cover the oven with meatballs, Italian-blended vegetables, and pasta. 2. Return the broth to a boil, reduce the heat to medium-low, and cook for around 10 minutes until the meatballs are hot and the pasta is tender. Garnish with parmesan cheese and ladle broth in bowls.

167.   Curried Zucchini Soup

(Ready in 45 minutes, Serve 6, Difficulty: Normal)
Nutrition per Serving: Calories: 227, Proteins: 1.8 g, Carbohydrates: 6.3 g, Fat: 5.2 g, Cholesterol: 0.5 mg, Sodium: 536.9 mg

Ingredients:

tablespoons of extra virgin olive oil large onion, halved and thinly sliced 1 tablespoon of curry powder Sea salt, to taste 4 small zucchinis, halved lengthwise and cut into 1-inch slices 1 quart of chicken stock

Instructions:

In a large pot, heat the oil. Stir in the onion, then add the curry powder and salt. Until the onion is tender, cook and stir. Stir in the zucchini mixture, then cook until tender. Pour the chicken stock into it. 2. Bring it to a boil. Cover, reduce heat to a low level and simmer for 20 minutes. 3. Remove soup from heat. Using a hand blender or transfer it to a blender in batches, then blend until almost smooth.

168.   Thick Cauliflower Soup

(Ready in 45 minutes, Serve 6, Difficulty: Easy)
Nutrition per Serving: Calories: 200, Proteins: 8 g, Carbohydrates: 25 g, Fat: 8 g.

Ingredients:

6 cups cauliflower, chopped 8 cups water ¾ teaspoon nutmeg 15 oz can white beans, drained and rinsed 3 cups chives, thinly chopped 2 cups onion, sliced 3 garlic cloves, minced tablespoon olive oil Salt to taste Pepper to taste

Instructions:

Heat oil, chives, and garlic for two minutes at a low heat. 2. Add cauliflower, nutmeg, and onion. Keep cooking for five more minutes 3. Incorporate water, and beans. Increase heat and let it boil. 4. Reduce heat and cook during 30 minutes on a medium-low heat, stirring occasionally. 5. Serve hot with bread.

169. Cheesy Keto Zucchini Soup

Preparation and **Cooking Time:** 20 minutes | **Servings:** 2

INGREDIENTS

½ medium onion, peeled and chopped 1 cup bone broth 1 tablespoon coconut oil 1½ zucchinis, cut into chunks ½ tablespoon nutrition al yeast Dash of black pepper ½ tablespoon parsley, chopped, for garnish ½ tablespoon coconut cream, for garnish

DIRECTIONS

Melt the coconut oil in a large pan over medium heat and add onions. Sauté for about 3 minutes and add zucchinis and bone broth. Reduce the heat to simmer for about 15 minutes and cover the pan. Add nutrition al yeast and transfer to an immersion blender. Blend until smooth and season with black pepper. Top with coconut cream and parsley to serve.

NUTRITION: Calories: 154 Carbs: 8.9g Fats: 8.1g Proteins: 13.4g Sodium: 93mg Sugar: 3.9g

170. Mint Avocado Chilled Soup

Preparation and **Cooking Time:** 15 minutes | **Servings:** 2

INGREDIENTS

romaine lettuce leaves 1 Tablespoon lime juice 1 medium ripe avocado 1 cup coconut milk, chilled 20 fresh mint leaves Salt to taste

DIRECTIONS Put all the ingredients in a blender and blend until smooth. Refrigerate for about 10 minutes and serve chilled.

NUTRITION: Calories: 432 Carbs: 16.1g Fats: 42.2g Proteins: 5.2g Sodium: 33mg Sugar: 4.5g

171. Spring Soup Recipe with Poached Egg

Preparation and **Cooking Time:** 20 minutes | **Servings:** 2

INGREDIENTS 2 eggs 2 tablespoons butter 4 cups chicken broth 1 head of romaine lettuce, chopped Salt, to taste

DIRECTIONS Boil the chicken broth and lower heat. Poach the eggs in the broth for about 5 minutes and remove the eggs. Place each egg into a bowl and add chopped romaine lettuce into the broth. Cook for about 10 minutes and ladle the broth with the lettuce into the bowls.

NUTRITION: Calories: 264 Carbs: 7g Fats: 18.9g Proteins: 16.1g Sodium: 1679mg Sugar: 3.4g

172. Swiss Chard Egg Drop Soup

Preparation and **Cooking Time:** 20 minutes | **Servings:** 4

INGREDIENTS

cups bone broth 2 eggs, whisked 1 teaspoon ground oregano 3 tablespoons butter 2 cups Swiss chard, chopped 2 tablespoons coconut aminos 1 teaspoon ginger, grated Salt and black pepper, to taste

DIRECTIONS Heat the bone broth in a saucepan and add whisked eggs while stirring slowly. Add the swiss chard, butter, coconut aminos, ginger, oregano and salt and black pepper. Cook for about 10 minutes and serve hot.

NUTRITION: Calories: 185 Carbs: 2.9g Fats: 11g Proteins: 18.3g Sodium: 252mg Sugar: 0.4g

173. Delicata Squash Soup

Preparation and **Cooking Time:** 45 minutes | **Servings:** 5

INGREDIENTS

1½ cups beef bone broth 1small onion, peeled and grated. ½ teaspoon sea salt ¼ teaspoon poultry seasoning 2small Delicata Squash, chopped 2 garlic cloves, minced 2tablespoons olive oil ¼ teaspoon black pepper 1 small lemon, juiced 5 tablespoons sour cream

DIRECTIONS Put Delicata Squash and water in a medium pan and bring to a boil. Reduce the heat and cook for about 20 minutes. Drain and set aside. Put olive oil, onions, garlic and poultry seasoning in a small sauce pan. Cook for about 2 minutes and add broth. Allow it to simmer for 5 minutes and remove from heat. Whisk in the lemon juice and transfer the mixture in a blender. Pulse until smooth and top with sour cream.

NUTRITION: Calories: 109 Carbs: 4.9g Fats: 8.5g Proteins: 3g Sodium: 279mg Sugar: 2.4g

174. Apple Pumpkin Soup

Preparation and **Cooking Time:** 10 minutes | **Servings:** 8

INGREDIENTS

1 apple, chopped 1 whole kabocha pumpkin, peeled, seeded and cubed 1 cup almond flour ¼ cup ghee 1 pinch cardamom powder 2 quarts water ¼ cup coconut cream 1 pinch ground black pepper

DIRECTIONS Heat ghee in the bottom of a heavy pot and add apples. Cook for about 5 minutes on a medium flame and add pumpkin. Sauté for about 3 minutes and add almond flour. Sauté for about 1 minute and add water. Lower the flame and cook for about 30 minutes. Transfer the soup into an immersion blender and blend until smooth. Top with coconut cream and serve.

NUTRITION: Calories: 186 Carbs: 10.4g Fats: 14.9g Proteins: 3.7g Sodium: 7mg Sugar: 5.4g

175.   Cauliflower and Thyme Soup

Preparation and **Cooking Time:** 30 minutes | **Servings:** 6

INGREDIENTS 2 teaspoonsthyme powder 1head cauliflower   3cupsvegetable stock ½ teaspoon matcha green tea powder 3tablespoonsolive oil Salt and black pepper, to taste 5garlic cloves, chopped

DIRECTIONS Put the vegetable stock, thyme and matcha powder to a large pot over medium-high heat and bring to a boil. Add cauliflower and cook for about 10 minutes. Meanwhile, put the olive oil and garlic in a small sauce pan and cook for about 1 minute. Add the garlic, salt and black pepper and cook for about 2 minutes. Transfer into an immersion blender and blend until smooth. Dish out and serve immediately.

NUTRITION: Calories: 79 Carbs: 3.8g Fats: 7.1g Proteins: 1.3g Sodium: 39mg Sugar: 1.5g

176.   Chicken Kale Soup

Preparation and **Cooking Time:** 6 hours 10 minutes | **Servings:** 6

INGREDIENTS

2 poundschicken breast, skinless 1/3cuponion 1tablespoonolive oil 14 ounceschicken bone broth ½ cup olive oil 4 cups chicken stock ¼ cup lemon juice 5ouncesbaby kale leaves Salt, to taste

DIRECTION S Season chicken with salt and black pepper. Heat olive oil over medium heat in a large skillet and add seasoned chicken. Reduce the temperature and cook for about 15 minutes. Shred the chicken and place in the crock pot. Process the chicken broth and onions in a blender and blend until smooth. Pour into crock pot and stir in the remaining ingredients. Cook on low for about 6 hours, stirring once while cooking.

NUTRITION: Calories: 261 Carbs: 2g Fats: 21g Proteins: 14.1g Sodium: 264mg Sugar: 0.3g

177.   Chicken Mulligatawny Soup

Preparation and **Cooking Time:** 30 minutes | **Servings:** 10

INGREDIENTS

1½ tablespoons curry powder 3 cups celery root, diced 2 tablespoons Swerve 10 cups chicken broth 5 cups chicken, chopped and cooked ¼ cup apple cider ½ cup sour cream ¼ cup fresh parsley, chopped 2 tablespoons butter Salt and black pepper, to taste

DIRECTIONS

Combine the broth, butter, chicken, curry powder, celery root and apple cider in a large soup pot. Bring to a boil and simmer for about 30 minutes. Stir in Swerve, sour cream, fresh parsley, salt and black pepper. Dish out and serve hot.

NUTRITION: Calories: 215 Carbs: 7.1g Fats: 8.5g Proteins: 26.4g Sodium: 878mg Sugar: 2.2g

178.   Traditional Chicken Soup

Preparation and **Cooking Time:** 1 hours 45 minutes | **Servings:** 6

INGREDIENTS

pounds chicken 4 quarts water 4 stalks celery 1/3 large red onion 1 large carrot 3 garlic cloves 2 thyme sprigs 2 rosemary sprigs Salt and black pepper, to taste

DIRECTIONS Put water and chicken in the stock pot on medium high heat. Bring to a boil and allow it to simmer for about 10 minutes. Add onion, garlic, celery, salt and pepper and simmer on medium low heat for 30 minutes. Add thyme and carrots and simmer on low for another 30 minutes. Dish out the chicken and shred the pieces, removing the bones. Return the chicken pieces to the pot and add rosemary sprigs. Simmer for about 20 minutes at low heat and dish out to serve.

NUTRITION: Calories: 357 Carbs: 3.3g Fats: 7g Proteins: 66.2g Sodium: 175mg Sugar: 1.1g

179.   Chicken Cabbage Soup

Preparation Time: 35 minutes | **Servings:** 8

INGREDIENTS   2celery stalks 2garlic cloves, minced 4 oz.butter 6 oz. mushrooms, sliced 2 tablespoons onions, dried and minced 1 teaspoon salt 8 cups chicken broth 1medium carrot 2 cups green cabbage, sliced into strips 2 teaspoons dried parsley ¼ teaspoon black pepper 1½ rotisserie chickens, shredded

DIRECTIONS Melt butter in a large pot and add celery, mushrooms, onions and garlic into the pot. Cook for about 4 minutes and add broth, parsley, carrot, salt and black pepper. Simmer for about 10 minutes and add cooked chicken and cabbage. Simmer for an additional 12 minutes until the cabbage is tender. Dish out and serve hot.

NUTRITION: Calories: 184 Carbs: 4.2g Fats: 13.1g Proteins: 12.6g Sodium: 1244mg Sugar: 2.1g

180. Keto BBQ Chicken Pizza Soup

Preparation Time: 1 hours 30 minutes | **Servings:** 6

INGREDIENT S 6 chicken legs 1 medium red onion, diced 4 garlic cloves 1 large tomato, unsweetened 4 cups green beans ¾ cup BBQ Sauce 1½ cups mozzarella cheese, shredded ¼ cup ghee 2 quarts water 2 quarts chicken stock Salt and black pepper, to taste Fresh cilantro, for garnishing

DIRECTIONS Put chicken, water and salt in a large pot and bring to a boil. Reduce the heat to medium-low and cook for about 75 minutes. Shred the meat off the bones using a fork and keep aside. Put ghee, red onions and garlic in a large soup and cook over a medium heat. Add chicken stock and bring to a boil over a high heat. Add green beans and tomato to the pot and cook for about 15 minutes. Add BBQ Sauce, shredded chicken, salt and black pepper to the pot. Ladle the soup into serving bowls and top with shredded mozzarella cheese and cilantro to serve.

NUTRITION: Calories: 449 Carbs: 7.1g Fats: 32.5g Proteins: 30.8g Sodium: 252mg Sugar: 4.7g

181. Spicy Halibut Tomato Soup

Preparation Time: 1 hours 5minutes | **Servings:** 8

INGREDIENTS
2 garliccloves, minced 1tablespoonolive oil ¼ cup fresh parsley, chopped 10anchoviescanned in oil, minced 6 cupsvegetable broth 1 teaspoonblack pepper 1 poundhalibut fillets, chopped 3 tomatoes, peeled and diced 1 teaspoonsalt 1 teaspoonred chili flakes

DIRECTIONS

Heat olive oil in a large stockpot over medium heat and add garlic and half of the parsley. Add anchovies, tomatoes, vegetable broth, red chili flakes, salt and black pepper and bring to a boil. Reduce the heat to medium-low and simmer for about 20 minutes. Add halibut fillets and cook for about 10 minutes. Dish

out the halibut and shred into small pieces. Mix back with the soup and garnish with the remaining fresh parsley to serve.

NUTRITION: Calories: 170 Carbs: 3g Fats: 6.7g Proteins: 23.4g Sodium: 2103mg Sugar: 1.8g

182. Fall Soup

Total Time: 40 minutes | Serves: 4

INGREDIENT S

1 carrot, chopped 1 leek, chopped 2 garlic cloves, minced 1 celery stalk, chopped 1 parsnip, chopped 1 potato, chopped 4 cups vegetable broth 3 cups chopped butternut squash 1 tsp dried thyme 2 tbsp olive oil Salt and black pepper to taste

DIRECTION S

Warm olive oil in a pot over medium heat and sauté leek, garlic, parsnip, carrot, and celery for 5-6 minutes until the veggies start to brown. Throw in squash, potato, broth, thyme, salt, and pepper. Bring to a boil, then decrease the heat and simmer for 20-30 minutes until the veggies soften. Transfer to a food processor and blend until you get a smooth and homogeneous consistency.

NUTRITION Per Serving: Calories 200, Fat 8.7g, Carbs 25.8g, Protein 7.2g

183. Sausage & Spinach Chickpea Soup

Total Time: 35 minutes | Serves: 6

INGREDIENTS 8 oz Italian sausage, sliced 1 (14-oz) can chickpeas, drained 4 cups chopped spinach 1 onion, chopped 1 carrot, chopped 1 red bell pepper, seeded and chopped 3 garlic cloves, minced 6 cups chicken broth 1 tsp dried oregano Salt and black pepper to taste 2 tbsp olive oil ½ tsp red pepper flakes

DIRECTION S Warm olive oil in a pot over medium heat. Sear the sausage for 5 minutes until browned. Set aside. Add carrot, onion, garlic, and bell pepper to the pot and sauté for 5 minutes until soft. Pour in broth, chickpeas, spinach, oregano, salt, pepper, and red flakes; let simmer for 5 minutes until the spinach softens. Bring the sausage back to the pot and cook for another minute. Serve warm.

NUTRITION Per Serving: Calories 473, Fat 21g, Carbs 46.7g, Protein 26.2g

184.   Veggie & Chicken Soup

Total Time: 35 minutes | Serves: 4

INGREDIENT S 1 cup mushrooms, chopped 2 tsp olive oil 1 large carrot, chopped 1 yellow onion, chopped 1 celery stalk, chopped 2 yellow squash, chopped 2 chicken breasts, cubed ½ cup chopped fresh parsley 4 cups chicken stock Salt and black pepper to taste

DIRECTION S Warm the oil in a skillet over medium heat. Place in carrot, onion, mushrooms, and celery and cook for 5 minutes. Stir in chicken and cook for 10 more minutes. Mix in squash, salt, and black pepper. Cook for 5 minutes, then lower the heat and pour in the stock. Cook covered for 10 more minutes. Divide between bowls and scatter with parsley. Serve immediately.

NUTRITION Per Serving: Calories 335, Fat 9g, Carbs 28g, Protein 33g

185.   Chicken Soup with Green Beans & Rice

Total Time: 45 minutes | Serves: 4

INGREDIENT S 4 cups chicken stock 2 tbsp olive oil ½ lb chicken breasts, cut into strips 1 celery stalk, chopped 2 garlic cloves, minced 1 yellow onion, chopped ½ cup white rice 1 egg, whisked ½ lemon, juiced 1 cup green beans, trimmed and chopped 1 cup carrots, chopped ½ cup dill, chopped Salt and black pepper to taste

DIRECTION S Warm the olive oil in a pot over medium heat and sauté onion, garlic, celery, carrots, and chicken for 6-7 minutes. Pour in stock and rice. Bring to a boil and simmer for 10 minutes. Stir in green beans, salt, and pepper and cook for another 15 minutes. Whisk the egg and lemon juice and pour into the pot. Stir and cook for 2 minutes. Serve warm.

NUTRITION Per Serving: Calories 270, Fat 19g, Carbs 20g, Protein 15g

186.   Turkey & Rice Egg Soup

Total Time: 40 minutes | Serves: 4

INGREDIENT S 1 lb turkey breasts, cubed ½ cup Arborio rice 1 onion, chopped 2 tbsp olive oil 1 celery stalk, chopped 1 carrot, sliced 1 egg 2 tbsp yogurt 1 tsp dried tarragon 1 tsp lemon zest 2 tbsp fresh parsley, chopped Salt and black pepper to taste

DIRECTION S Heat olive oil in a pot over medium heat and sauté the onion, celery, turkey, and carrot for 6-7 minutes, stirring occasionally. Stir in the rice for 1-2 minutes, pour in 4 cups of water, and season with salt and pepper. Bring the soup to a boil. Lower the heat and simmer for 20 minutes until thoroughly cooked. In a bowl, beat the egg with yogurt until well combined. Remove 1 cup of the hot soup broth with a spoon and add slowly to the egg mixture, stirring constantly. Pour the whisked mixture into the pot and stir in salt, black pepper, tarragon, and lemon zest. Garnish with parsley and serve.

NUTRITION Per Serving: Calories 303, Fat 10.6g, Carbs 28.6g, Protein 23.3g

187.   Oregano Chicken & Barley Soup

Total Time: 40 minutes | Serves: 4

INGREDIENT S

1 lb boneless chicken thighs ¼ cup pearl barley 2 tbsp olive oil 1 red onion, chopped 2 cloves garlic, minced 4 cups chicken broth ¼ tsp oregano ½ lemon, juiced ¼ tsp parsley ¼ cup fresh scallions, chopped Salt and black pepper to taste

DIRECTION S

Heat the olive oil in a pot over medium heat and sweat the onion and garlic for 2-3 minutes until tender. Place in chicken thighs and cook for 5-6 minutes, stirring often. Pour in chicken broth and barley and bring to a boil. Then lower the heat and simmer for 5 minutes. Remove the chicken and shred it with two forks. Return to the pot and add in barley, lemon, oregano, and parsley. Simmer for 20-22 more minutes. Stir in shredded chicken and adjust the seasoning. Divide between 4 bowls and top with chopped scallions. Serve hot.

NUTRITION Per Serving: Calories 373, Fat 17g, Carbs 14.2g, Protein 39.4g

188.   Slow Cooked Hot Lentil Soup

Total Time: 8 hours and 10 minutes | Serves: 6

INGREDIENT S

1 cup dry lentils 2 carrots, sliced 1 yellow onion, chopped 2 celery stalks, chopped 2 garlic cloves, minced 14 oz canned tomatoes, chopped 1 tbsp red pepper flakes 6 cups vegetable stock ½ tsp cumin Salt and black pepper to taste ¼ cup oregano, chopped 2 tbsp lime juice

DIRECTION S

Place lentils, tomatoes, onion, celery, carrots, garlic, vegetable stock, cumin, red pepper flakes, salt, and pepper in your slow cooker. Place the lid cook on

Low for 8 hours. Stir in oregano and lime juice and serve right away.

NUTRITION Per Serving: Calories 280, Fat 2g, Carbs 49g, Protein 18g

189. Italian Cavolo Nero Soup

Total Time: 35 minutes | Serves: 4

INGREDIENT S 2 tbsp olive oil 1 lb cavolo nero, torn 1 cup canned chickpeas, drained Salt and black pepper to taste 1 celery stalk, chopped 1 onion, chopped 1 carrot, chopped 14 oz canned tomatoes, chopped 2 tbsp rosemary, chopped 4 cups vegetable stock

DIRECTION S Warm the olive oil in a pot over medium heat and cook onion, celery, and carrot for 5 minutes. Stir in cavolo nero, salt, pepper, tomatoes, rosemary, chickpeas, and vegetable stock and simmer for 20 minutes. Serve warm.

NUTRITION Per Serving: Calories 200, Fat 9g, Carbs 13g, Protein 5g

190. Vegetable Soup

Total Time: 55 minutes | Serves: 4

INGREDIENT S 2 tbsp olive oil 1 yellow onion, chopped 2 garlic cloves, minced 1 carrot, chopped 1 zucchini, chopped 1 yellow squash, peeled and cubed 2 tbsp parsley, chopped ¼ fennel bulb, chopped 30 oz canned cannellini beans, drained 2 cups veggie stock ¼ tsp dried thyme Salt and black pepper to taste 1 cup green beans ¼ cup Parmesan cheese, grated

DIRECTION S Warm the olive oil in a pot over medium heat and cook onion, garlic, carrot, squash, zucchini, and fennel for 5 minutes. Stir in cannellini beans, veggie stock, 4 cups of water, thyme, salt, and pepper and bring to a boil; cook for 10 minutes. Put in broccoli and cook for another 10 minutes. Serve sprinkled with Parmesan cheese and parsley.

NUTRITION Per Serving: Calories 310, Fat 12g, Carbs 18g, Protein 11g

191. Tasty Zuppa Toscana

Total Time: 25 minutes | Serves: 6

INGREDIENT S

2 tbsp olive oil 1 yellow onion, chopped 4 garlic cloves, minced 1 celery stalk, chopped 1 carrot, chopped 15 oz canned tomatoes, chopped 1 zucchini, chopped 6 cups vegetable stock 2 tbsp tomato paste 15 oz canned white beans, drained and rinsed 5 oz

Tuscan kale 1 tbsp basil, chopped Salt and black pepper to taste

DIRECTIONS

Warm the olive oil in a pot over medium heat and cook garlic and onion for 3 minutes. Stir in celery, carrot, tomatoes, zucchini, stock, tomato paste, white beans, kale, salt, and pepper and bring to a simmer. Cook for 10 minutes. Serve topped with basil.

NUTRITION Per Serving: Calories 480, Fat 9g, Carbs 77g, Protein 28g

192. Spinach & Lentil Soup

Total Time: 55 minutes | Serves: 4

INGREDIENT S

2 tbsp olive oil 1 yellow onion, chopped 2 celery stalks, chopped 1 carrot, sliced 2 tbsp parsley, chopped 2 garlic cloves, minced 2 tbsp ginger, grated 1 tsp turmeric powder 2 tsp sweet paprika 1 tsp cinnamon powder ½ cup red lentils 1 cup spinach, torn 14 oz canned tomatoes, crushed 4 cups chicken stock Salt and black pepper to taste

DIRECTION S Warm the olive oil in a pot over medium heat and sauté onion, ginger, garlic, celery, and carrot for 5 minutes. Stir in turmeric powder, sweet paprika, cinnamon powder, red lentils, tomatoes, chicken stock, salt, and pepper and bring to a boil. Simmer for 15 minutes. Stir in spinach for 5 minutes until the spinach is wilted. Sprinkle with parsley and serve.

NUTRITION Per Serving: Calories 250, Fat 8g, Carbs 33g, Protein 15g

193. Super Bean & Celery

Soup **Total Time:** 50 minutes | Serves: 4

INGREDIENT S

2 tbsp olive oil 2 shallots, chopped 1 potato, chopped 5 celery sticks, chopped 1 carrot, chopped ½ tsp dried oregano 1 bay leaf 30 oz canned white beans, drained 2 tbsp tomato paste 4 cups chicken stock

DIRECTION S Warm the olive oil in a pot over medium heat and cook shallots, celery, carrot, bay leaf, and oregano for 5 minutes. Stir in white beans, tomato paste, potato, and chicken stock and bring to a boil. Cook for 20 minutes. Remove the bay leaf. Serve.

NUTRITION Per Serving: Calories 280, Fat 17g, Carbs 16g, Protein 8g

194. Power Green

Soup **Total Time:** 20 minutes | Serves: 4

INGREDIENTS 1 tbsp olive oil 1 white onion, chopped ½ cup Greek yogurt 1 celery stalk, chopped 4 cups vegetable stock 2 cups green peas 2 tbsp mint leaves, chopped 1 cup spinach Salt and black pepper to taste

DIRECTION S Warm the olive oil in a pot over medium heat and cook onion and celery for 4 minutes. Add in vegetable stock, green peas, spinach, salt, and pepper and bring to a boil. Simmer for 4 minutes. Take off the heat and let cool the soup for a few minutes. Blend the soup with an immersion blender until smooth. Apportion the soup among bowls and garnish with a swirl of Greek yogurt. Sprinkle with chopped mint and serve.

NUTRITION Per Serving: Calories 300, Fat 12g, Carbs 28g, Protein 5g

195. Tomato Beef Soup

Total Time: 1 hour | Serves: 4

INGREDIENTS

2 tbsp olive oil ½ lb beef stew meat, cubed 1 celery stalk, chopped 1 tsp fennel seeds 1 tsp hot paprika 1 carrot, chopped 1 onion, chopped Salt and black pepper to taste 2 garlic cloves, chopped 4 cups beef stock ½ tsp dried cilantro 1 tsp dried oregano 14 oz canned tomatoes, chopped 2 tbsp parsley, chopped

DIRECTION S Warm the olive oil in a pot over medium heat and cook beef meat, onion, and garlic for 10 minutes, stirring occasionally. Stir in celery, carrots, fennel seeds, paprika, salt, pepper, cilantro, and oregano for 3 minutes. Pour in beef stock and tomatoes and bring to a boil. Cook for 40 minutes. Sprinkle with parsley. Serve immediately.

NUTRITION Per Serving: Calories 350, Fat 16g, Carbs 16g, Protein 38g

196. Easy Vegetable

Soup **Total Time:** 40 minutes | Serves: 4

INGREDIENT S

2 tbsp olive oil 2 potatoes, peeled and cubed 1 celery stalk, chopped 1 zucchini, chopped 1 small head broccoli, chopped 1 onion, chopped 1 carrot, cubed 1 tsp dried rosemary ½ tsp cayenne pepper 4 cups vegetable stock Salt and black pepper to taste 1 tbsp chives, chopped

DIRECTION S

Warm the olive oil in a pot over medium heat and sauté onion, celery, and carrot for 5 minutes. Add in rosemary, cayenne pepper, potatoes, and zucchini and sauté for another 5 minutes. Pour in the vegetable stock and bring to a simmer. Cook for 20 minutes. Adjust the seasoning and add in the broccoli; cook for 5-8 minutes. Sprinkle with chives. Serve immediately.

NUTRITION Per Serving: Calories 260, Fat 12g, Carbs 18g, Protein 13g

197. Chicken & Eggplant

Soup **Total Time:** 40 minutes | Serves: 4

INGREDIENT S

2 tbsp butter ¼ tsp celery seeds 2 cups eggplants, cubed Salt and black pepper to taste 1 red onion, chopped 2 garlic cloves, minced 1 red bell pepper, chopped 1 red chili pepper 2 tbsp parsley, chopped 2 tbsp oregano, chopped 4 cups chicken stock 1 lb chicken breasts, cubed 1 cup half and half 1 egg yolk

DIRECTION S Melt butter in a pot over medium heat and sauté chicken, garlic, and onion for 10 minutes. Put in bell pepper, eggplant, salt, pepper, red chili pepper, celery seeds, oregano, and chicken stock and bring to a simmer. Cook for 20 minutes. Whisk egg yolk, half and half, and 1 cup of the soup in a bowl and pour gradually into the pot. Stir and sprinkle with parsley. Serve immediately.

NUTRITION Per Serving: Calories 320, Fat 18g, Carbs 21g, Protein 16g

198. Cold Prawn

Soup **Total Time:** 15 minutes | Serves: 6

INGREDIENT S 3 tbsp olive oil 1 cucumber, chopped 3 cups tomato juice 3 roasted red peppers, chopped 2 tbsp balsamic vinegar 1 garlic clove, minced Salt and black pepper to taste ½ tsp cumin 1 lb prawns, peeled and deveined 1 tsp thyme, chopped

DIRECTION S

In a food processor, blitz tomato juice, cucumber, red peppers, 2 tbsp of olive oil, vinegar, cumin, salt, pepper, and garlic until smooth. Remove to a bowl and transfer to the fridge for 10 minutes. Warm the remaining oil in a pot over medium heat and sauté prawns, salt, pepper, and thyme for 4 minutes on all sides. Let cool. Ladle the soup into individual bowls and serve topped with prawns.

NUTRITION Per Serving: Calories 270, Fat 12g, Carbs 13g, Protein 7g

199. Spinach & Orzo

Soup **Total Time:** 20 minutes | Serves: 4
INGREDIENT S
2 tbsp butter 3 cups spinach ½ cup orzo 4 cups chicken broth 1 cup feta cheese, crumbled Salt and blac k pepper to taste ½ tsp dried oregano 1 onion, chopped 2 garlic cloves, minced 1 cup mushrooms, sliced

DIRECTIONS Melt butter in a pot over medium heat and sauté onion, garlic, and mushrooms for 5 minutes until tender. Add in chicken broth, orzo, salt, pepper, and oregano. Bring to a boil and reduce the heat to a low. Continue simmering for 10 minutes, partially covered. Stir in spinach and continue to cook until the spinach wilts, about 3-4 minutes. Ladle into individual bowls and serve garnished with feta cheese. Enjoy!
NUTRITION Per Serving: Calories 370, Fat 11g, Carbs 44g, Protein 23g

200. Spicy Chicken Soup with Beans

Total Time: 40 minutes | Serves: 6
INGREDIENT S
3 tbsp olive oil 3 garlic cloves, minced 1 onion, chopped 3 tomatoes, chopped 4 cups chicken stock 1 lb chicken breasts, cubed 1 red chili pepper, chopped 1 tbsp fennel seeds, crushed 14 oz canned white beans, drained 1 lime, zested and juiced Salt and black pepper to taste 1 tbsp parsley, chopped
DIRECTION S
Warm the olive oil in a pot over medium heat. Cook the onion and garlic, adding a splash of water, for 10 minutes until aromatic. Add in the chicken and chili pepper and sit-fry for another 6-8 minutes. Put in tomatoes, chicken stock, beans, lime zest, lime juice, salt, pepper, and fennel seeds and bring to a boil; cook for 30 minutes. Serve warm.
NUTRITION Per Serving: Calories 670, Fat 18g, Carbs 74g, Protein 56g

201. Leftover Lamb & Mushroom Soup

Total Time: 40 minutes | Serves: 4
INGREDIENTS
2 carrots, chopped 1 red onion, chopped 2 tbsp olive oil 2 celery stalks, chopped 2 garlic cloves, minced Salt and black pepper to taste 1 tbsp thyme, chopped 4 cups vegetable stock 1 cup white mushrooms, sliced 8 oz leftover lamb, shredded 14 oz canned chickpeas, drained 2 tbsp cilantro, chopped
DIRECTION S
Warm the olive oil in a pot over medium heat and cook onion, celery, mushrooms, carrots, and thyme for 5 minutes until tender. Stir in vegetable stock and lamb and bring to a boil. Reduce the heat to low and simmer for 20 minutes. Mix in chickpeas and cook for an additional 5 minutes. Ladle your soup into individual bowls. Top with cilantro and serve hot.
NUTRITION Per Serving: Calories 300, Fat 12g, Carbs 23g, Protein 15g
Spring Soup with Poached Egg
Preparation and **Cooking Time:** 20 minutes | **Servings:** 2
INGREDIENTS 32 oz vegetable broth 2 eggs 1 head romaine lettuce, chopped Salt, to taste
DIRECTIONS
Bring the vegetable broth to a boil and reduce the heat. Poach the eggs for 5 minutes in the broth and remove them into 2 bowls.
Stir in romaine lettuce into the broth and cook for 4 minutes. Dish out in a bowl and serve hot.
NUTRITION: Calories: 158 Carbs: 6.9g Fats: 7.3g Proteins: 15.4g Sodium: 1513mg Sugar: 3.3g

202. Easy Butternut Squash Soup

Preparation and **Cooking Time:** 1 hour 45 minutes | **Servings:** 4
INGREDIENTS
1 small onion, chopped 4 cups chicken broth 1 butternut squash 3 tablespoons coconut oil Salt, to taste Nutmeg and pepper, to taste
DIRECTIONS
Put oil and onions in a large pot and add onions. Sauté for about 3 minutes and add chicken broth and butternut squash. Simmer for about 1 hour on medium heat and transfer into an immersion blender. Pulse until smooth and season with salt, pepper and nutmeg. Return to the pot and cook for about 30 minutes. Dish out and serve hot.
NUTRITION: Calories: 149 Carbs: 6.6g Fats: 11.6g Proteins: 5.4g Sodium: 765mg Sugar: 2.2g

203. Cauliflower, leek & bacon soup

Preparation and **Cooking Time:** 10 minutes | **Servings:** 4

INGREDIENTS

cups chicken broth ½ cauliflower head, chopped 1 leek, chopped Salt and black pepper, to taste 5 bacon strips

DIRECTIONS

Put the cauliflower, leek and chicken broth into the pot and cook for about 1 hour on medium heat. Transfer into an immersion blender and pulse until smooth. Return the soup into the pot and microwave the bacon strips for 1 minute. Cut the bacon into small pieces and put into the soup. Cook on for about 30 minutes on low heat. Season with salt and pepper and serve.

NUTRITION: Calories: 185 Carbs: 5.8g Fats: 12.7g Proteins: 10.8g Sodium: 1153mg Sugar: 2.4g

204. Mushroom Spinach Soup

Preparation and **Cooking Time:** 25 minutes | **Servings:** 4

INGREDIENTS

1cupspinach,cleaned and chopped 100 g mushrooms,chopped 1 onion 6 garlic cloves ½ teaspoon red chili powder Salt and black pepper, to taste 3 tablespoons buttermilk 1 teaspoon almond flour 2 cups chicken broth 3 tablespoons butter ¼ cup fresh cream for garnish

DIRECTIONS

Heat butter in a pan and add onions and garlic. Sauté for about 3 minutes and add spinach, salt and red chili powder. Sauté for about 4 minutes and add mushrooms. Transfer into a blender and blend to make a puree. Return to the pan and add buttermilk and almond flour for creamy texture. Mix well and simmer for about 2 minutes. Garnish with fresh cream and serve hot.

NUTRITION: Calories: 160 Carbs: 7g Fats: 13.3g Proteins: 4.7g Sodium: 462mg Sugar: 2.7g

205. Broccoli Soup

Preparation and **Cooking Time:** 10 minutes | **Servings:** 6

INGREDIENTS

3 tablespoons ghee 5 garlic cloves 1 teaspoon sage ¼ teaspoon ginger 2 cups broccoli 1 small onion 1 teaspoon oregano ½ teaspoon parsley Salt and black

pepper, to taste 6 cups vegetable broth 4 tablespoons butter

DIRECTIONS

Put ghee, onions, spices and garlic in a pot and cook for 3 minutes. Add broccoli and cook for about 4 minutes. Add vegetable broth, cover and allow it to simmer for about 30 minutes. Transfer into a blender and blend until smooth. Add the butter to give it a creamy delicious texture and flavor

NUTRITION: Calories: 183 Carbs: 5.2g Fats: 15.6g Proteins: 6.1g Sodium: 829mg Sugar: 1.8g

206. Keto French Onion Soup

Preparation and **Cooking Time:** 40 minutes | **Servings:** 6

INGREDIENT S 5 tablespoons butter 500 g brown onion medium 4 drops liquid stevia 4 tablespoons olive oil 3 cups beef stock

DIRECTIONS

Put the butter and olive oil in a large pot over medium low heat and add onions and salt. Cook for about 5 minutes and stir in stevia. Cook for another 5 minutes and add beef stock. Reduce the heat to low and simmer for about 25 minutes. Dish out into soup bowls and serve hot.

NUTRITION: Calories: 198 Carbs: 6g Fats: 20.6g Proteins: 2.9g Sodium: 883mg Sugar: 1.7g

207. Homemade Thai Chicken Soup

Preparation and **Cooking Time:** 8 hours 25 minutes | **Servings:** 12

INGREDIENTS

1 lemongrass stalk, cut into large chunks 5 thick slices of fresh ginger 1 whole chicken 20 fresh basil leaves 1 lime, juiced 1 tablespoon salt

DIRECTIONS

Place the chicken, 10 basil leaves, lemongrass, ginger, salt and water into the slow cooker. Cook for about 8 hours on low and dish out into a bowl. Stir in fresh lime juice and basil leaves to serve.

NUTRITION: Calories: 255 Carbs: 1.2g Fats: 17.6g Proteins: 25.2g Sodium: 582mg Sugar: 0.1g

208. Chicken Veggie Soup

Preparation and **Cooking Time:** 20 minutes | **Servings:** 6

INGREDIENTS

chicken thighs 12 cups water 1 tablespoon adobo seasoning 4 celery ribs 1 yellow onion 1½ teaspoons whole black peppercorns 6 sprigs fresh parsley 2 teaspoons coarse sea salt 2 carrots 6 mushrooms, sliced 2 garlic cloves 1 bay leaf 3 sprigs fresh thyme

DIRECTIONS

Put water, chicken thighs, carrots, celery ribs, onion, garlic cloves and herbs in a large pot. Bring to a boil and reduce the heat to low. Cover the pot and simmer for about 30 minutes. Dish out the chicken and shred it, removing the bones. Put the bones back into the pot and simmer for about 20 minutes. Strain the broth, discarding the chunks and put the liquid back into the pot. Bring it to a boil and simmer for about 30 minutes. Put the mushrooms in the broth and simmer for about 10 minutes. Dish out to serve hot.

NUTRITION: Calories: 250 Carbs: 6.4g Fats: 8.9g Proteins: 35.1g Sodium: 852mg Sugar: 2.5g

209. Buffalo Ranch Chicken Soup

Preparation and **Cooking Time:** 40 minutes | **Servings:** 4

INGREDIENTS

2 tablespoons parsley 2 celery stalks, chopped 6 tablespoons butter 1 cup heavy whipping cream 4 cups chicken, cooked and shredded 4 tablespoons ranch dressing ¼ cup yellow onions, chopped 8 oz cream cheese 8 cups chicken broth 7 hearty bacon slices, crumbled

DIRECTIONS

Heat butter in a pan and add chicken. Cook for about 5 minutes and add 1½ cups water. Cover and cook for about 10 minutes. Put the chicken and rest of the ingredients into the saucepan except parsley and cook for about 10 minutes. Top with parsley and serve hot.

NUTRITION: Calories: 444 Carbs: 4g Fats: 34g Proteins: 28g Sodium: 1572mg Sugar: 2g

210. Chicken Noodle Soup

Preparation and **Cooking Time:** 30 minutes | **Servings:** 6

INGREDIENTS

1 onion, minced 1 rib celery, sliced 3 cups chicken, shredded 3 eggs, lightly beaten 1 green onion, for garnish 2 tablespoons coconut oil 1 carrot, peeled and thinly sliced 2 teaspoons dried thyme 2½ quarts homemade bone broth ¼ cup fresh parsley, minced Salt and black pepper, to taste

DIRECTION S

Heat coconut oil over medium-high heat in a large pot and add onions, carrots, and celery. Cook for about 4 minutes and stir in the bone broth, thyme and chicken. Simmer for about 15 minutes and stir in parsley. Pour beaten eggs into the soup in a slow steady stream. Remove soup from heat and let it stand for about 2 minutes. Season with salt and black pepper and dish out to serve.

NUTRITION: Calories: 226 Carbs: 3.5g Fats: 8.9g Proteins: 31.8g Sodium: 152mg Sugar: 1.6g

211. Green Chicken Enchilada Soup

Preparation Time: 20 minutes | Servings: 5

INGREDIENTS

oz. cream cheese, softened ½ cup salsa verde 1 cup cheddar cheese, shredded 2 cups cooked chicken, shredded 2 cups chicken stock

DIRECTIONS

Put salsa verde, cheddar cheese, cream cheese and chicken stock in an immersion blender and blend until smooth. Pour this mixture into a medium saucepan and cook for about 5 minutes on medium heat. Add the shredded chicken and cook for about 5 minutes. Garnish with additional shredded cheddar and serve hot.

NUTRITION: Calories: 265 Carbs: 2.2g Fats: 17.4g Proteins: 24.2g Sodium: 686mg Sugar: 0.8g

212. Salmon Stew Soup

Preparation Time: 25 minutes | Servings: 5

INGREDIENTS

4 cups chicken broth 3 salmon fillets, chunked 2 tablespoons butter 1 cup parsley, chopped 3 cups Swiss chard, roughly chopped 2 Italian squash, chopped 1 garlic clove, crushed ½ lemon, juiced Salt and black pepper, to taste 2 eggs

DIRECTIONS

Put the chicken broth and garlic into a pot and bring to a boil. Add salmon, lemon juice and butter in the pot and cook for about 10 minutes on medium heat. Add Swiss chard, Italian squash, salt and pepper and cook for about 10 minutes. Whisk eggs and add to the pot, stirring continuously. Garnish with parsley and serve.

NUTRITION: Calories: 262 Carbs: 7.8g Fats: 14g Proteins: 27.5g Sodium: 1021mg Sugar: 1.2g

213. Italian Chicken & Veggie Soup

Total Time: 30 minutes | Serves: 4

INGREDIENT S 1 (14-oz) can diced tomatoes ½ pound chicken breasts, cubed 4 cups chicken broth 2 carrots, chopped 1 onion, chopped 1 red bell pepper, seeded and chopped 1 fennel bulb, chopped 2 garlic cloves, minced ½ tsp paprika 1 cup mushrooms, sliced 1 tbsp Italian seasoning 2 tbsp olive oil Salt and black pepper to taste

DIRECTION S Warm olive oil in a pot over medium heat. Place in chicken and brown for 5 minutes. Set aside. Add in onion, carrots, bell pepper, and fennel, sauté for 5 minutes until softened. Throw in garlic and paprika and cook for 30 seconds. Mix in tomatoes, mushrooms, Italian seasoning, broth, chicken, salt, and pepper. Bring to a boil, then decrease the heat and simmer for 20 minutes. Serve warm.

NUTRITION Per Serving: Calories 293, Fat 14.2g, Carbs 18.5g, Protein 24.4g

214. Rosemary Soup with Roasted Vegetables

Total Time: 45 minutes | Serves: 4

INGREDIENT S 2 carrots, sliced 3 tbsp olive oil 3 sweet potatoes, sliced 1 celery stalk, sliced 1 tsp chopped rosemary 4 cups vegetable broth Salt and black pepper to taste Grated Parmesan cheese

DIRECTION S Preheat oven to 400°F. Mix carrots, sweet potatoes, and celery in a bowl. Drizzle with olive oil and toss. Sprinkle with rosemary, salt, and pepper. Arrange on a lined with parchment paper sheet and bake for 30 minutes or until the veggies are tender and golden brown. Remove from the oven and let cool slightly. Place the veggies and some broth in a food processor and pulse until smooth; work in batches. Transfer to a pot over low heat and ad d in the remaining broth. Cook just until heated through. Serve topped with Parmesan cheese.

NUTRITION Per Serving: Calories 203, Fat 10g, Carbs 23g, Protein 2g

215. Spicy Lentil Soup

Total Time: 30 minutes | Serves: 4

INGREDIENT S

1 cup lentils, rinsed 1 onion, chopped 2 carrots, chopped 1 potato, cubed 1 tomato, chopped 4 garlic cloves , minced 4 cups vegetable broth 2 tbsp olive oil ½ tsp chili powder Salt and black pepper to taste 2 tbsp fresh parsley, chopped

DIRECTION S Warm olive oil in a pot over medium heat. Add in onion, garlic, and carrots and sauté for 5-6 minutes until tender. Mix in lentils, broth, salt, pepper, chili powder, potato, and tomato. Bring to a boil, lower the heat and simmer for 15-18 minutes, stirring often. Top with parsley and serve.

NUTRITION Per Serving: Calories 331, Fat 9g, Carbs 44.3g, Protein 19g

216. Basil Meatball Soup

Total Time: 35 minutes | Serves: 6

INGREDIENT S

1 (14-oz) can chopped tomatoes, drained ½ cup rice, rinsed 12 oz ground beef 2 shallots, chopped 1 tbs p dried thyme 1 carrot, chopped 1 tsp garlic powder 2 tbsp olive oil 5 garlic cloves, minced 6 cups chicken broth ¼ cup chopped fresh basil leaves Salt and black pepper to taste

DIRECTION S Combine ground beef, shallots, garlic powder, thyme, salt, and pepper in a bowl. Make balls out of the mixture and reserve. Warm the olive oil in a pot over medium heat and sauté the garlic and carrot for 2 minutes. Mix in meatballs, rice, tomatoes, broth, salt, and pepper and bring to a boil. Lower the heat and simmer for 18 minutes. Top with basil before serving.

NUTRITION Per Serving: Calories 265, Fat 9.8g, Carbs 18.8g, Protein 24.2g

217. Basil Tomato & Roasted Pepper Soup

Total Time: 30 minutes | Serves: 4

INGREDIENT S 1 cup roasted bell peppers, chopped 3 tomatoes, cored and halved 2 cloves garlic, whole 1 yellow onion, quartered 1 celery stalk, chopped 1 carrot, shredded ½ tsp ground cumin 1 chili pepper, seeded 2 tbsp olive oil 4 cups vegetable broth ½ tsp red pepper flakes, crushed 2 tbsp fresh basil, chopped Salt and black pepper to taste ¼ cup crème fraîche

DIRECTION S Arrange the Roma tomatoes, garlic, onion, and peppers on a roasting pan. Drizzle olive oil over your vegetables. Heat olive oil in a pot over medium heat and sauté onion, garlic, celery, and carrots for 3-5 minutes until tender. Stir in chili pepper and cumin for 1-2 minutes. Pour in roasted bell peppers and tomatoes, stir, then add in the vegetable broth. Season with salt and pepper. Bring to a boil and reduce the heat; simmer for 10 minutes.

Using an immersion blender, purée the soup until smooth. Sprinkle with red pepper flakes and basil. Serve topped with crème fraîche.
NUTRITION Per Serving: Calories 164, Fat 11.6g, Carbs 9.8g, Protein 6.5g

218. Pork & Vegetable Soup

Total Time: 40 minutes | Serves: 4
INGREDIENT S
2 tbsp olive oil 1 onion, chopped 2 garlic cloves, minced 1 pork loin, chopped 1 cup mushrooms, chopped 1 carrot, chopped 1 celery stalk, chopped Salt and black pepper to taste 14 oz canned tomatoes, drained 4 cups vegetable stock ½ tsp nutmeg, ground 2 tsp parsley, chopped
DIRECTION S Warm the olive oil in a pot over medium heat and cook pork meat, onion, and garlic for 5 minutes. Put in mushrooms, carrots, salt, pepper, tomatoes, vegetable stock, and nutmeg and bring to a boil. Cook for 25 minutes. Sprinkle with parsley.
NUTRITION Per Serving: Calories 240, Fat 6g, Carbs 22g, Protein 7g

219. Herbed Bean Soup

Total Time: 50 minutes | Serves: 6
INGREDIENTS
2 tbsp olive oil 6 cups veggie stock 1 cup celery, chopped 1 cup carrots, chopped 1 yellow onion, chopped 2 garlic cloves, minced ½ cup navy beans, soaked ½ tsp chopped parsley ½ tsp paprika 1 tsp thyme Salt and black pepper to taste
DIRECTION S
Warm olive oil in a saucepan and sauté onion, garlic, carrots, and celery for 5 minutes, stirring occasionally. Stir in paprika, thyme, salt, and pepper for 1 minute. Pour in chicken broth and navy beans. Bring to a boil, then reduce the heat and simmer for 40 minutes covered. Sprinkle with basil and serve hot.
NUTRITION Per Serving: Calories 270, Fat 18g, Carbs 24g, Protein 12g

220. Quick Chicken & Vermicelli Soup

Total Time: 25 minutes | Serves: 4
INGREDIENT S
2 tbsp olive oil 1 carrot, chopped 1 leek, chopped ½ cup vermicelli 4 cups chicken stock 2 cups kale, chopped 2 chicken breasts, cubed 1 cup orzo ¼ cup lemon juice 2 tbsp parsley, chopped Salt and black pepper to taste
DIRECTION S
Warm the olive oil in a pot over medium heat and sauté leek and chicken for 6 minutes. Stir in carrot and chicken stock and bring to a boil. Cook for 10 minutes. Add in vermicelli, kale, orzo, and lemon juice and continue cooking for another 5 minutes. Adjust the seasoning with salt and pepper and sprinkle with parsley. Ladle into soup bowls and serve.
NUTRITION Per Serving: Calories 310, Fat 13g, Carbs 17g, Protein 13g

221. Cannellini Bean & Feta Cheese Soup

Total Time: 30 minutes | Serves: 4
INGREDIENTS
4 oz feta cheese, crumbled 1 cup collard greens, torn into pieces 2 cups canned cannellini beans, rinsed 2 tbsp olive oil 1 fennel bulb, chopped 1 carrot, chopped ½ cup spring onions, chopped ½ tsp dried rosemary ½ tsp dried basil 1 garlic clove, minced 4 cups vegetable broth 2 tbsp tomato paste Salt and black pepper to taste
DIRECTION S In a pot over medium heat, warm the olive oil. Add in fennel, garlic, carrot, and spring onions and sauté until tender, about 2-3 minutes. Stir in tomato paste, rosemary, and basil and cook for 2 more minutes. Pour in vegetable broth and cannellini beans.
Bring to a boil, then lower the heat, and simmer for 15 minutes. Add in collard greens and cook for another 2-3 minutes until wilted. Adjust the seasoning with salt and pepper. Top with feta cheese and serve.
NUTRITION Per Serving: Calories 519, Fat 15.4g, Carbs 64.6g, Protein 32.3g

222. Italian Sausage & Seafood Soup

Total Time: 30 minutes | Serves: 4
INGREDIENT S ½ lb shrimp, raw and deveined 2 tbsp butter 3 Italian sausages, sliced 1 red onion, chopped 1 ½ cups clams 1 carrot, chopped 1 celery stalk, chopped 2 garlic cloves, minced 1 (14.5-oz) canned tomatoes 1 tsp dried basil 1 tsp dried dill 4 cups chicken broth 2 tbsp olive oil 4 tbsp cornflour 2 tbsp lemon juice 2 tbsp fresh cilantro, chopped Salt and black pepper to taste

DIRECTION S Melt the butter in a pot over medium heat and brown the sausage; set aside. Heat the olive oil in the same pot and add in cornflour; cook for 4 minutes. Add in the onion, garlic, carrot, and celery and stir-fry them for 3 minutes. Stir in tomatoes, basil, dill, and chicken broth. Bring to a boil. Lower the heat and simmer for 5 minutes. Mix in the reserved sausages, salt, black pepper, clams, and shrimp and simmer for 10 minutes. Discard any unopened clams. Share into bowls and sprinkle with lemon juice. Serve warm garnished with fresh cilantro.
NUTRITION Per Serving: Calories 619, Fat 42.6g, Carbs 26.6g, Protein 32.5g

223. Cauliflower Soup with Pancetta Croutons

Total Time: 50 minutes | Serves: 4
INGREDIENT S
4 oz pancetta, cubed 2 tbsp olive oil 1 cauliflower head, cut into florets 1 yellow onion, chopped Salt an d black pepper to taste 4 cups chicken stock 1 tsp mustard powder 2 garlic cloves, minced ½ cup mozzarella cheese, shredded
DIRECTIONS
Place a saucepan over medium heat and add in the pancetta. Cook it until crispy, about 4 minutes, and set aside. Add olive oil, onion, and garlic to the pot and cook for 3 minutes. Pour in chicken stock, cauliflower, mustard powder, salt, and pepper and cook for 20 minutes.
Using an immersion blender, purée the soup and stir in the mozzarella cheese. Serve immediately topped with pancetta croutons.
NUTRITION Per Serving: Calories 250, Fat 18g, Carbs 42g, Protein 14g

224. Cheesy Tomato Soup

Total Time: 45 minutes | Serves: 4
INGREDIENT S
2 tbsp olive oil 2 lb tomatoes, halved 2 garlic cloves, minced 1 onion, chopped Salt and black pepper to taste 4 cups chicken stock ½ tsp red pepper flakes ½ cup basil, chopped ½ cup Pecorino cheese, grated
DIRECTIONS
Preheat the oven to 380°F. Place the tomatoes in a baking tray, drizzle with olive oil, and season with salt and pepper. Roast in the oven for 20 minutes. Warm the remaining olive oil in a pot over medium heat and sauté onion for 3 minutes. Put in roasted tomatoes,

garlic, chicken stock, and red pepper flakes and bring to a boil. Simmer for 15 minutes. Using an immersion blender, purée the soup and stir in Pecorino cheese. Serve right away topped with basil.
NUTRITION Per Serving: Calories 240, Fat 11g, Carbs 16g, Protein 8g

225. Pork Meatball Soup

Total Time: 35 minutes | Serves: 4
INGREDIENTS
2 tbsp olive oil ½ cup white rice ½ lb ground pork Salt and black pepper to taste 2 garlic cloves, minced 1 onion, chopped ½ tsp dried thyme 4 cups beef stock ½ tsp saffron powder 14 oz canned tomatoes, crushed 1 tbsp parsley, chopped
DIRECTION S In a bowl, mix ground pork, rice, salt, and pepper with your hands. Shape the mixture into ½-inch balls; set aside. Warm the olive oil in a pot over medium heat and cook the onion and garlic for 5 minutes. Pour in beef stock, thyme, saffron powder, and tomatoes and bring to a boil. Add in the pork balls and cook for 20 minutes. Adjust the seasoning with salt and pepper. Serve sprinkled with parsley.
NUTRITION Per Serving: Calories 380, Fat 18g, Carbs 29g, Protein 18g

226. Turkey & Cabbage

Soup **Total Time:** 40 minutes | Serves: 4
INGREDIENT S
2 tbsp olive oil ½ lb turkey breast, cubed 2 leeks, sliced 4 spring onions, chopped 1 green cabbage head, shredded 4 celery sticks, chopped 4 cups vegetable stock ½ tsp sweet paprika ½ tsp ground nutmeg Salt and black pepper to taste
DIRECTION S Warm the olive oil in a pot over medium heat and brown turkey for 4 minutes, stirring occasionally. Add in leeks, spring onions, and celery and cook for another minute. Stir in cabbage, vegetable stock, sweet paprika, nutmeg, salt, and pepper and bring to a boil. Cook for 30 minutes. Serve immediately.
NUTRITION Per Serving: Calories 320, Fat 16g, Carbs 25g, Protein 19g

227. Green Lentil & Ham

Soup **Total Time:** 30 minutes | Serves: 6
INGREDIENTS
½ lb ham, cubed 1 onion, chopped 2 tbsp olive oil 2 tsp parsley, dried 1 potato, chopped 3 garlic cloves,

chopped Salt and black pepper to taste 1 carrot, chopped ½ tsp paprika ½ cup green lentils, rinsed 4 cups vegetable stock 3 tbsp tomato paste 2 tomatoes, chopped

DIRECTION S

Warm the olive oil in a pot over medium heat and cook ham, onion, carrot, and garlic for 4 minutes. Stir in tomato paste, paprika, and tomatoes for 2-3 minutes. Pour in lentils, vegetable stock, ham, and potato and bring to a boil. Cook for 18-20 minutes. Adjust the seasoning with salt and pepper and sprinkle with parsley. Serve warm.

NUTRITION Per Serving: Calories 270, Fat 12g, Carbs 25g, Protein 15g

228.   Lamb & Spinach

Soup **Total Time:** 50 minutes | Serves: 4

INGREDIENT S

2 tbsp olive oil ½ lb lamb meat, cubed 3 eggs, whisked 4 cups beef broth 5 spring onions, chopped 2 tbsp mint, chopped 2 lemons, juiced Salt and black pepper to taste 1 cup baby spinach

DIRECTIONS

Warm the olive oil in a pot over medium heat and cook lamb for 10 minutes, stirring occasionally. Add in spring onions and cook for another 3 minutes. Pour in beef broth, salt, and pepper and simmer for 30 minutes. Whisk eggs with lemon juice and some soup and pour into the pot along with the spinach and cook for an additional 5 minutes. Sprinkle with mint and serve immediately.

NUTRITION Per Serving: Calories 290, Fat 29g, Carbs 3g, Protein 6g

229.   Lemon Chicken

Soup **Total Time:** 40 minutes | Serves: 4

INGREDIENT S

2 tbsp olive oil 1 onion, chopped 2 garlic cloves, minced 1 celery stalk, chopped 1 carrot, chopped 4 cups chicken stock Salt and black pepper to taste ¼ cup lemon juice 1 chicken breast, cubed ½ cup stelline pasta 6 mint leaves, chopped

DIRECTION S Warm the olive oil in a pot over medium heat and sauté onion, garlic, celery, and carrot for 5 minutes until tender. Add in the chicken and cook for another 4-5 minutes, stirring occasionally. Pour in chicken stock and bring to a boil; cook for 10 minutes. Add in the stelline past and let simmer for 10 minutes. Stir in lemon juice and adjust the seasoning with salt and pepper. Sprinkle

with mint and ladle the soup into bowls. Serve immediately.

NUTRITION Per Serving: Calories 240, Fat 12g, Carbs 15g, Protein 13g

230.   Spanish Chorizo & Bean

Soup **Total Time:** 45 minutes | Serves: 4

INGREDIENT S 2 tbsp olive oil 1 lb Spanish chorizo, sliced 1 carrot, chopped 1 yellow onion, chopped 1 celery stalk, chopped 2 garlic cloves, minced ½ lb kale, chopped 4 cups chicken stock 1 cup canned Borlotti beans, drained 1 tsp rosemary, dried Salt and black pepper to taste ½ cup Manchego cheese, grated

DIRECTION S Warm the olive oil in a large pot over medium heat and cook sausage for 5 minutes or until the fat is rendered and the chorizo is browned. Add in onion and continue to cook for another 3 minutes until soft and translucent. Stir in garlic and let it cook for 30-40 seconds until fragrant. Lastly, add the carrots and celery and cook for 4-5 minutes or so until tender. Now, pour in the chicken stock, drained and washed beans, rosemary, salt, and pepper and bring to a boil. Reduce the heat to low, cover the pot and simmer for 30 minutes. Stir periodically, checking to make sure there is enough liquid. Five minutes before the end, add the kale. Adjust the seasoning. Ladle your soup into bowls and serve topped with Manchego cheese.

NUTRITION Per Serving: Calories 580, Fat 27g, Carbs 38g, Protein 27g

231.   Turkish Chicken Soup with Buckwheat

Total Time: 40 minutes | Serves: 6

INGREDIENT S

1 tbsp olive oil 1 lb chicken breasts, cubed Salt and black pepper to taste 2 celery stalks, chopped 1 carrot, chopped 1 red onion, chopped 6 cups chicken stock ½ cup parsley, chopped ½ cup buckwheat 1 tsp lime juice 1 lime, sliced

DIRECTION S

Warm the olive oil in a pot over medium heat. Season chicken breasts with salt and pepper and cook for 8 minutes. Stir in onion, carrot, and celery and sauté for another 3 minutes or until soft and aromatic. Put in chicken stock and buckwheat and bring to a boil. Reduce the heat to low. Let it simmer for about 20 minutes and add in lime juice. Sprinkle with parsley. Ladle your soup into individual bowls and serve warm with gremolata toast and the lime slices. Yummy!

NUTRITION Per Serving: Calories 320, Fat 9g, Carbs 18g, Protein 24g

232.   Cauliflower-Cheese Soup

(Ready in 45 minutes, Serve 4, Difficulty: Normal)

Nutrition per Serving: Calories: 138, Protein: 15.7 g, Carbohydrates: 25.9 g, Fat: 24.7 g, Cholesterol: 74.9 mg, Sodium: 367.6 mg.

Ingredients:

¾ cup of water 1 cup of chopped cauliflower 1 cup of cubed potatoes ½ cup of finely chopped celery ½ cup of diced carrots ¼ cup of chopped onion ¼ cup of butter ¼ cup of all-purpose flour 3 cups of milk Salt and pepper, to taste 4 ounces of shredded cheddar cheese

Instructions:

Combine the water, cauliflower, carrots, potatoes, celery, and onion in a large saucepan. It should be boiled for 5-10 minutes, or until tender. Only put aside. 2. Over medium pressure, melt the butter in a separate saucepan. Add the flour, then simmer for 2 minutes. 3. Remove from the heat, and stir in the milk gradually. Return to the heat and simmer until the mixture thickens.

With the cooking liquid, stir in the vegetables and season with salt and pepper. Remove from the heat and whisk in the cheese until melted.

233.   Sweet Potato, Carrot, Apple, and Red Lentil Soup

(Ready in 1 hour and 10 minutes, Serve 6, Difficulty: Normal)

Nutrition per Serving: Calories: 232, Protein: 9 g, Carbohydrates: 52.9 g, Fat: 9 g, Cholesterol: 21.6 mg, Sodium: 876.3 mg.

Ingredients:

¼ cup of butter 2 large sweet potatoes, peeled and chopped 3 large carrots, peeled and chopped apple, peeled, cored, and chopped 1 onion, chopped ½ cup of red lentils ½ teaspoon of minced fresh ginger ½ teaspoon of ground black pepper 1 teaspoon of salt ½ teaspoon of ground cumin ½ teaspoon of chili powder ½ teaspoon of paprika 4 cups of vegetable broth Plain yogurt

Instructions:

Melt the butter over medium-high heat in a big heavy-bottomed pot. In the pot, combine the chopped sweet potatoes, carrots, apple, and onion.

Stir and cook the apples and vegetables for about 10 minutes before the onions are translucent. 2. In a pot with the apple and vegetable mixture, stir the lentils, ginger, ground black pepper, cinnamon, chili powder, paprika, and vegetable broth. Bring the soup to a boil over high heat, then reduce the heat to medium-low, cover and simmer for about 30 minutes until the lentils and vegetables are soft. 3. Pour the soup into a blender, working in batches, filling the pitcher no more than halfway full. With a folded kitchen towel, keep the blender's lid down and start the blender carefully, using a few short pulses to transfer the soup before leaving it to puree. Purée until smooth and pour into a clean pot in batches. Alternately, right in the cooking pot, you should use a stick blender to puree the broth. 4. Place the pureed soup back in the cooking pot. Bring back over medium-high heat, around 10 minutes, to a simmer. To thin the soup to your desired consistency, add water as needed. For garnish, serve with yogurt. 5. Instead of yogurt as a garnish, this soup is also well served with crumbled feta cheese.

234.   Vegetarian Kale Soup

(Ready in 55 minutes, Serve 8, Difficulty: Normal)

Nutrition per Serving: Calories: 277, Protein: 9.6 g, Carbohydrates: 50.9 g, Fat: 4.5 g, Cholesterol: 0 mg, Sodium: 372.2 mg.

Ingredients:

2 tablespoons of olive oil yellow onion, chopped tablespoons of chopped garlic 1 bunch of kale, stems removed and leaves chopped 8 cups of water 6 cubes of vegetable bouillon (such as Knorr®) 1(15 ounces) can of diced tomatoes 6 white potatoes, peeled and cubed 2(15 ounces) cans of cannellini beans (drained if desired) 1 tablespoon of Italian seasoning tablespoons of dried parsley Salt and pepper, to taste

Instructions:

In a large soup pot, heat the olive oil and cook the onion and garlic until soft. Stir in the kale and cook for about 2 minutes, until wilted. Stir in the water, stir up the water 2. Tomatoes, potatoes, beans, vegetable bouillon, Italian seasoning, and parsley. Simmer the soup for 25 minutes on medium heat or until the potatoes are fully cooked. To taste, season with salt and pepper.

235. Butternut and Acorn Squash Soup

(Ready in 1 hour and 20 minutes, Serve 8, Difficulty: Hard)

Nutrition per Serving: Calories: 266, Protein: 5.1 g, Carbohydrates: 33.8 g, Fat: 14.5 g, Cholesterol: 42.2 mg, Sodium: 139.3 mg.

Ingredients:

butternut squash, halved and seeded 1 acorn squash, halved and seeded tablespoons of butter ¼ cup of chopped sweet onion 1 quart of chicken broth 1 cup of packed brown sugar 1(8 ounces) package of cream cheese, softened ½ teaspoon of ground black pepper ½ teaspoon of ground cinnamon to taste Fresh parsley, for garnish

Instructions:

Preheat the oven to 350 degrees Fahrenheit (176 degrees Celsius). Place the side-cut squash halves in a baking dish. Bake until tender or 45 minutes. Remove from the heat and slightly cool. Scoop the skins with the pulp and discard. 2. Melt the butter over medium heat in a skillet, and sauté the onion until it is tender. 3. Mix the squash pulp, onion, cream cheese, broth, brown sugar, pepper, and cinnamon in a blender or food processor until smooth. This can be carried out in several batches. 4. Transfer the soup over medium heat to a pot and cook, occasionally stirring, until thoroughly heated. Garnish with parsley and warm to serve.

236. Ukrainian Red Borscht Soup

(Ready in 1 hour and 5 minutes, Serve 10, Difficulty: Normal)

Nutrition per Serving: Calories: 257, Protein: 10.1 g, Carbohydrates: 24.4 g, Fat: 13.8 g, Cholesterol: 31 mg, Sodium: 626.3 mg.

Ingredients:

1(16 ounces) package of pork sausage 3 medium beets, peeled and shredded 3 carrots, peeled and shredded 3 medium baking potatoes, peeled and cubed tablespoon of vegetable oil 1 medium onion, chopped 1(6 ounces) can of tomato paste ¾ cup of water ½ medium head cabbage, cored and shredded 1(8 ounces) can of diced tomatoes, drained cloves of garlic, minced Salt and pepper, to taste 1 teaspoon of white sugar, or to taste For Topping: ½ cup of sour cream For Garnish: 1 tablespoon of chopped fresh parsley

Instructions:

Crumble (if using the sausage over medium-high heat into a skillet. Cook and stir until it is not pink anymore. Remove and set aside from the heat. 2. Fill a large pot with water halfway (about 2 quarts) and bring it to a boil. Stir in the sausage, then cover the pot. Return to a boil. Add the beets, and cook until their color is gone. Add the carrots and potatoes, and cook for about 15 minutes, until tender. Add the cabbage, the diced tomatoes, and the can. 3. Over medium heat, heat the oil in a skillet. Add the onion, then cook until it's tender. Combine the tomato paste and water until well mixed. To the pot, transfer. To the soup, add the raw garlic, cover, and turn the heat off. Let them stand for 5 minutes. Taste, and then season with salt, sugar, and pepper. 4. Ladle it into serving bowls and if desired, garnish it with sour cream and fresh parsley.

237. Hearty Corn and Pumpkin Soup

(Ready in 50 minutes, Serve 8, Difficulty: Normal)

Nutrition per Serving: Calories: 288, Protein: 7.1 g, Carbohydrates: 44.3 g, Fat: 11.1 g, Cholesterol: 7.2 mg, Sodium: 1819.6 mg.

Ingredients: 1/3 cup of olive oil 2 leeks, white and light green parts only, thinly sliced 2 carrots, peeled and diced 9 cups of chicken broth 5 small red potatoes, diced 1½ teaspoons of salt ¼ teaspoon of ground cloves Ground black pepper, to taste 2(16 ounces) cans of pumpkin puree 1(16 ounces) package of frozen whole-kernel corn ½ cup of whole milk tablespoon of minced fresh parsley, or to taste

Instructions: Over medium heat, heat the olive oil in a large pot. In hot oil, cook and stir the leeks and carrots until softened, for 5-10 minutes. 2. Stir the chicken broth into the leek mixture and bring it to a boil. Add the potatoes, salt, cloves, and pepper, and cook for about 15 minutes, until the potatoes are tender. 3. In a large bowl, pour in the pumpkin puree. Stir 1 cup of the mixed broth and potatoes into the pumpkin. 4. In a large pot, pour the pumpkin mixture, corn, and milk into the chicken broth mixture. Stir to combine and simmer, at least 5 minutes, until heated through and flavors blend. Sprinkle with parsley on individual servings.

238. Carrot and Ginger Soup

(Ready in 55 minutes, Serve 6, Difficulty: Normal)
Nutrition per Serving:Calories: 246, Protein: 3.5 g, Carbohydrates: 33.8 g, Fat: 12.8 g, Cholesterol: 20.4 mg, Sodium: 171.7 mg.

Ingredients: ½ medium butternut squash 2 tablespoons of olive oil onion, diced 453 g of carrots, peeled and diced cloves of garlic, crushed or to taste 1(2 inches) piece of fresh ginger, peeled and thinly sliced cups of water Salt and pepper, to taste 1 pinch of ground cinnamon ¼ cup of heavy cream (Optional)

Instructions: The oven should be preheated to 350 degrees Fahrenheit (176 degrees Celsius). Scoop the seeds from ½ of the butternut squash and place the cut side down on a greased baking sheet. Bake in the oven for 30-40 minutes or until tender. Allow to cool, then with a large spoon, scoop the squash flesh out of the skin and set aside. Discard the skin. 2. Over medium heat, heat the olive oil in a large saucepan or soup pot. Add the chopped onion and garlic and cook until the onion is translucent, stirring well. Add the squash, carrots, and ginger and pour in the water. Bring to a boil and cook until the carrots and ginger are tender, for at least 20 minutes or until tender. 3. In a mixer, or with an immersion blender, purée the mixture. If necessary, add boiling water to thin it but keep in mind that this is meant to be a thick creamy soup. Send the soup back to the tub, and heat through it.

Use salt, pepper, and cinnamon to season. 4. Ladle into serving bowls and as a garnish, if desired, pour a small swirl of cream over the end.

239. Squash and Apple Soup

(Ready in 35 minutes, Serve 6, Difficulty: Easy)
Nutrition per Serving: Calories: 140, Protein: 3.1 g, Carbohydrates: 28.6 g, Fat: 2.8 g, Cholesterol: 4.8 mg, Sodium: 31.8 mg.

Ingredients:
2 teaspoons of butter onion, chopped 453 g of butternut squash, peeled and chopped apples, peeled and chopped 1 small potato, peeled and chopped 1 teaspoon of grated fresh ginger root 1 pinch of white pepper cups of water ¼ cup of apple cider 1 teaspoon of packed brown sugar ½ cup of plain yogurt 1 tablespoon of finely chopped toasted pecans

Instructions:

Cook the stew beef, onion, and celery in a large saucepan over medium-high heat for 5 minutes or until the meat is browned on all sides. 2. Add the bouillon, parsley, carrots, ground black pepper, and pasta with water and eggs. 3. Bring it to a boil, bring it to low heat, and cook for 30 minutes

240. Caramelized Butternut Squash Soup

(Ready in 50 minutes, Serve 1, Difficulty: Normal)
Nutrition per Serving: Calories: 189, Protein: 2.9 g, Carbohydrates: 24.9 g, Fat: 10.3 g, Cholesterol: 22.9 mg, Sodium: 788.4 mg.

Ingredients:
3 tablespoons of extra-virgin olive oil 1360 g of butternut squash, peeled and cubed large onion, sliced tablespoons of butter 1 tablespoon of sea salt 1 teaspoon of freshly-cracked white pepper cups of chicken broth, or more as needed ¼ cup of honey ½ cup of heavy whipping cream 1 pinch of ground nutmeg, or more to taste Salt, to taste Ground white pepper, to taste

Instructions:

In a large pot, heat olive oil over high heat. Cook and stir the squash until thoroughly browned, about 10 minutes, in hot oil. Stir in the squash onion, sugar, sea salt, and cracked white pepper, cook and stir until the onions are fully tender and begin to brown for about 10 minutes. 2. Over the mixture, add chicken broth and honey, bring to a boil, reduce heat to medium-low and simmer for around 5 minutes until the squash is tender. 3. Pour the mixture no more than half full into a blender. Cover and keep the lid in place and pulse a few times before mixing. In batches, purée until smooth. 4. Stir in the soup to serve with the milk, nutmeg, cinnamon, and ground white pepper.

241. Winter Root Vegetable Soup

(Ready in 1 hour and 35 minutes, Serve 6, Difficulty: Normal)
Nutrition per Serving: Calories: 132, Protein: 5.2 g, Carbohydrates: 40.7 g, Fat: 18 g, Cholesterol: 22.7 mg, Sodium: 1786.4 mg.

Ingredients:
3 parsnips, peeled and cut into ½-inch pieces 3 carrots, peeled and cut into ½-inch pieces celery root, peeled and cut into ½-inch pieces turnips, quartered 1 sweet potato, peeled and cut into ½-inch pieces 1(907 g) butternut squash, peeled and cut into ½-

inch pieces ¼ cup of olive oil 1 teaspoon of kosher salt ½ teaspoon of ground black pepper tablespoons of butter stalk of celery, diced ½ sweet onion, diced 1 quart of vegetable broth ½ cup of half-and-half cream Salt and ground black pepper, to taste
Instructions

Preheat the oven to 425 degrees Fahrenheit (218 degree Celsius). 2. In a large roasting pan, combine the turnips, carrots, turnips, sweet potato, celery root, and butternut squash. Season with one teaspoon of kosher salt and 1/2 teaspoon of pepper and spray with olive oil. Toss vegetables to spread seasonings equally. 3. Roast in the preheated oven for 30-45 minutes, stirring after 15 minutes until the vegetables are easily pierced with a fork. 4. Meanwhile, over medium heat, melt the butter in a big pot or Dutch oven. Stir in the onion and celery, cook and stir until the onion is tender and translucent, about 5 minutes. Pour in the bouillon of vegetables and put to a boil, uncovered. 5. Combine the roasted vegetables and begin to cook for 10 minutes. Use an immersion blender to puree the broth. 6. Add half and half, and if necessary, season with salt and pepper. Add more vegetable broth if the soup gets too thick.

242.   Butternut Vegetable Soup

(Ready in 1 hour and 45 minutes, Serve 10, Difficulty: Hard)
Nutrition per Serving: Calories: 187, Protein: 6.4 g, Carbohydrates: 27.3 g, Fat: 6.6 g, Sodium: 820.2 mg.

Ingredients:
¼ cup of vegetable oil cup of finely diced onion teaspoons of minced garlic large carrots, thinly sliced 2 cups of peeled and cubed butternut squash 12 cups of vegetable broth 2 red potatoes, cubed ½ teaspoon of dried thyme 1 teaspoon of salt ½ teaspoon of ground black pepper cups of finely chopped kale leaves 1(16 ounces) can of great northern beans, rinsed and drained
Instructions:

Heat the vegetable oil over medium heat in a big Dutch oven. Stir in the garlic and onion, cook and stir until the onion is tender and translucent, around 5 minutes. Stir in the butternut squash and carrots, cook, and stir for about 15 minutes before the squash starts to brown. 2. Pour the broth. Bring to a boil, stir in the red potatoes, thyme, salt, and pepper. Reduce the heat and boil for about 45 minutes until the vegetables are tender. Stir in the kale and the large

northern beans and boil for about 10 minutes until the kale is tender. 3. In a mixer, pour about 3 cups of the broth, filling the pitcher no more than halfway full (you may have to do this in two batches). With a folded kitchen towel, keep the blender's lid down and start the blender carefully, using a few short pulses to transfer the soup before leaving it to puree. 4. To the soup pot, return the pureed part of the soup, leaving the remaining soup chunky. Alternately, right in the boiling pot, you should use a stick blender to partly puree the soup.

243.   Spicy Chipotle Sweet Potato Soup

(Ready in 55 minutes, Serve 8, Difficulty: Normal)
Nutrition per Serving: Calories: 113, Protein: 5.2 g, Carbohydrates: 48.7 g, Fat: 15.7 g, Cholesterol: 33 mg, Sodium: 501.9 mg.

Ingredients:
2 tablespoons of olive oil large yellow onion, chopped 1587 g of sweet potatoes, peeled and cut into 2-inch chunks 4 ½ cups of vegetable broth, or as needed 1(7 ounces) can of chipotle peppers in adobo sauce, drained ½ cup of heavy cream limes, juiced Salt, to taste 1 cup of sour cream ½ cup of chopped fresh cilantro, or to taste
Instructions: Heat the olive oil over medium heat in a large saucepan or Dutch oven, cook and stir the onion in the hot oil until softened, for 3-5 minutes. 2. Add the sweet potatoes, bring to a boil, and enough vegetable broth to cover the sweet potatoes. Reduce the heat, cover the saucepan partially, and boil until around 30 minutes or until the sweet potatoes are soft enough for a fork to pierce easily. 3. Stir in the sweet potato mixture with the chipotle peppers. 4. Using an immersion blender to process the sweet potato mixture until the soup is smooth. Whisk in the broth with heavy cream and lime juice until smooth and cooked through, and season with salt. 5. Serve each serving of soup served with 2 teaspoons of sour cream and a cilantro sprinkle.

244.   Green Tomato and Bacon Soup

(Ready in 1 hour and 10 minutes, Serve 6, Difficulty: Normal)
Nutrition per Serving: Calories: 212, Protein 7.1 g, Carbohydrates: 12.1 g, Fat: 5.7 g, Cholesterol: 13.4 mg, Sodium: 655 mg.

Ingredients: 8 slices of bacon, cut into bite-size pieces small red onion, chopped, or to taste cloves of garlic, minced, or to taste 5 cups of chopped green tomatoes cups of vegetable broth ½ teaspoon of celery salt, or to taste 1 bay leaf, or to taste Freshly ground black pepper, to taste

Instructions: Place the bacon over medium-low heat in a stockpot, cook and stir until the bacon starts to brown, around 5 minutes. Stir in the bacon with the onion and garlic cloves 2. Cook and stir for about 10 minutes, until the onion is tender. Mix the bacon-onion combination with green tomatoes, celery salt, vegetable broth, bay leaf, and black pepper. 3. Bring it to a boil. Reduce the heat and simmer for about 40 minutes, until the tomatoes are tender.

Chapter 5:

Vegetarian Recipes

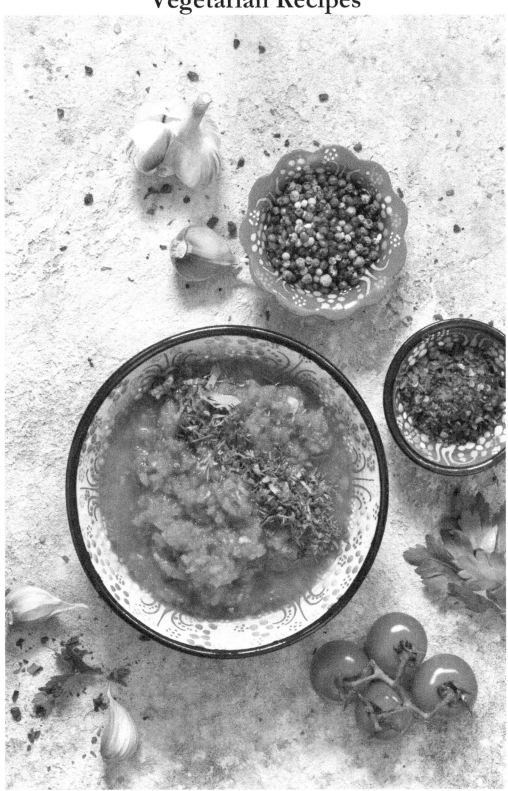

245.   Herby Raita

Preparation Time: 10 Minutes
Cooking Time: 0 Minutes
Servings: 2-4
Ingredients:
1 Large-sized cucumber, shredded
½ Tsp. of sea salt
1 Cup of Greek yogurt
¼ Cup of freshly chopped mint
1 Tsp. of lemon juice
¼ Tsp. of freshly ground black pepper
Directions:
Mix the cucumber with ¼ teaspoon of salt in a sieve and leave to drain for 15 minutes. Shake to release any excess liquid and transfer to a kitchen towel. Squeeze out as much liquid as possible using the paper towel.
Place the cucumber into a medium bowl, then stir in the remaining ingredients until well combined.
Place in the refrigerator for at least 2 hours to keep it fresh. It is best consumed with spicy foods to relieve the spiciness.
Nutrition:
Calories: 69 kcal Protein: 4.33g
Fat: 3.66g Carbohydrates: 4.93g

246.   Balsamic Vinaigrette

Preparation Time: 10 Minutes
Cooking Time: 0 Minutes
Servings: 2-4
Ingredients:
½ Cup of extra-virgin olive oil
½ Cup of rice vinegar
Tsp. of Dijon mustard
1 Clove of freshly minced garlic
1 Tbsp. of honey or maple syrup
1 Tsp. of sea or kosher salt
¼ Tsp. of freshly ground black pepper

Directions:
Place all ingredients in a mason jar and cover tightly. Shake well until all ingredients are combined.
Keep in the refrigerator for at least 30 minutes before serving to keep it fresh.
Serve with your favorite salad or as your meat marinate.
Nutrition:
Calories: 147 kcal
Protein: 1.85g Fat: 13.21g
Carbohydrates: 4.02g

247.   Strawberry Poppy Seed

Preparation Time: 10 Minutes
Cooking Time: 0 Minutes
Servings: 2-4
Ingredients:
1/3 Cup of honey
¼ Cup of raspberry vinegar
Tbsp. of freshly squeezed orange juice
½ Tsp. of onion powder
¼ Tsp. of sea salt
¼ Tsp. of ground ginger
1/3 cup of extra-virgin olive oil
½ Tsp. of poppy seeds
Directions:
Place all ingredients, except the poppy seeds and oil, into a blender. Blend until smooth and creamy. Then, gradually put the oil into the mixture until emulsified. Add in the poppy seeds and stir well.
Place the mixture in a mason jar, put it in the refrigerator before serving. Keep for up to 3 days. Serve with your garden salads.
Nutrition:
Calories: 167 kcal
Protein: 1.84g
Fat: 9.35g
Carbohydrates: 18.89g

248.   Creamy Avocado Dressing

Preparation Time: 10 Minutes
Cooking Time: 0 Minutes
Servings: 2-4
Ingredients:
2 Small or one large-sized avocado, pitted and chopped
½ Cup of extra-virgin olive oil
1 Tsp. of honey or maple syrup
1 Clove of garlic, chopped
Tbsp. of red wine vinegar
2 Tsp. of lemon or lime juice
3 Tbsp. of chopped parsley
Onion powder
Some Kosher salt and ground black pepper
Directions:
Put all the ingredients together into a blender, except the oil. As the ingredients are blended, gradually add the oil into the mixture. Blend until smooth or becomes liquidy.

Use as a vegetable or fruit salad dressing. Put in the refrigerator for up to 5 days.

Nutrition:

Calories: 300 kcal Protein: 4.09g

Fat: 27.9g Carbohydrates: 11.41g

249.   Apple and Tomato Dipping Sauce

Preparation Time: 10 Minutes

Cooking Time: 0 Minutes

Servings: 2-4

Ingredients:

1 Tbsp. of extra-virgin olive oil

1 Large-sized shallot, diced

1 Tbsp. natural tomato paste

1 Garlic clove, finely chopped

½ Tsp. of sea salt

¼ Tsp. of freshly ground black pepper

1/8 Tsp. of ground cloves

3 Medium-sized apples, roughly chopped

3 Medium-sized tomatoes, roughly chopped

¼ Cup of cider vinegar

1 Tbsp. of maple syrup

Directions:

Put oil into a huge saucepan and heat it up over medium heat.

Add shallot and cook until light brown for about 2 minutes.

Mix in the tomato paste, garlic, salt, pepper, and cloves for about 30 seconds. Then add in the apples, tomatoes, vinegar, and maple syrup.

Bring to a boil, then reduce the heat to let it simmer for about 30 minutes. Let cool for another 20 minutes before placing the mixture into the blender. Blend the mixture until smooth.

Keep in a mason jar or an airtight container; refrigerate for up to 5 days.

Serve it on a burger or with fries.

Nutrition:

Calories: 142 kcal Protein: 3g

Fat: 3.46g Carbohydrates: 26.93g

250.   Dairy-Free   Creamy Turmeric

Preparation Time: 10 minutes

Cooking Time: 0 minutes

Servings: 2-4

Ingredients:

½ Cup of tahini

½ Cup of extra-virgin olive oil

2 Tbsp. of lemon juice

2 Tsp. of honey

1 Tbsp. of turmeric powder

Some sea salt and pepper

Directions:

In a bowl, whisk all ingredients until well combined. Store in a mason jar and refrigerate for up to 5 days.

Nutrition:

Calories: 328 kcal

Protein: 7.3g

Fat: 29.36g

Carbohydrates: 12.43g

251.   Homemade Ranch

Preparation Time: 10 Minutes

Cooking Time: 0 Minutes

Servings: 2-4

Ingredients:

½ Cup of natural mayonnaise, without preservatives

¼ Cup of Greek yogurt

2 Tsp. of dried chives

½ Tsp. of dried dill

½ Tsp. of dried parsley

½ Tsp. of garlic powder

½ Tsp. of onion powder

¼ Tsp. Kosher salt

1/8 Tsp. Freshly ground black pepper

¾ Cup of non-dairy milk

Directions:

Put all the ingredients together except the milk into a medium bowl. Whisk together until well combined. Add in the milk and mix well.

Pour in a mason jar or an airtight container. Serve immediately or refrigerate for up to 2 hours to keep it fresh. Place in the fridge for up to 5 days.

Serve with your favorite garden or fruit salad.

Nutrition:

Calories: 482 kcal

Protein: 3.55g

Fat: 51.98g

Carbohydrates: 1.63g

252.   Soy With Honey and Ginger Glaze

Preparation Time: 10 Minutes

Cooking Time: 0 Minutes

Servings: 2-4

Ingredients:

¼ Cup of honey

2 Tbsp. gluten-free soy sauce

1 Tbsp. of rice vinegar

1 Tsp. of freshly grated ginger

Directions:

Place all the ingredients together into a small bowl and whisk well.

Serve with your favorite vegetables, chickens, or seafood.

Keep the glaze in a mason jar, tightly covered, and refrigerate for up to 4 days.

Nutrition:

Calories: 90 kcal

Protein: 2.32g

Fat: 1.54g

Carbohydrates: 17.99g

253. Tahini Dip

Preparation Time: 10 Minutes

Cooking Time: 0 Minutes

Servings: 2-4

Ingredients:

1 Small clove of garlic, grated or finely minced (this is optional)

¼ Cup of tahini

1 Tbsp. of apple cider vinegar

1 Tbsp. of freshly squeezed lemon juice

1 Tbsp. of tamari

1 Tsp. of finely grated ginger, or ½ Tsp. of ground ginger

½ Tsp. of maple syrup

1 Tsp. of turmeric

1/3 Cup of water

Directions:

Blend or whisk all ingredients together. Put the dressing in an airtight container, then refrigerate for about five days.

Enjoy!

Nutrition:

Calories: 120 kcal

Protein: 4.77g

Fat: 9.63g

Carbohydrates: 5.12g

254. Homemade Lemon Vinaigrette

Preparation Time: 10 Minutes

Cooking Time: 0 Minutes

Servings: 2-4

Ingredients:

½ Tsp. of lemon zest

2 Tbsp. of freshly squeezed lemon juice

1 Tsp. of honey or maple syrup

½ Tsp. of Dijon mustard, without preservatives

¼ Tsp. of sea salt

3 Tbsp. of extra-virgin olive oil

Freshly ground black pepper

Directions:

Whisk all the ingredients together except olive oil and black pepper in a small bowl. Then gradually add three tablespoons of olive oil while constantly whisking until well combined. Add some ground black pepper to taste.

Put in a mason jar and refrigerate for up to 3 days. Serve with your favorite garden salads.

Nutrition:

Calories: 68 kcal

Protein: 1.69g

Fat: 6.06g

Carbohydrates: 1.71g

255. Creamy Raspberry Vinaigrette

Preparation Time: 10 Minutes

Cooking Time: 0 Minutes

Servings: 2-4

Ingredients:

2 Tbsp. of raspberry vinegar

2 Tbsp. of honey or maple syrup

1 Tbsp. of Greek yogurt

1 Tbsp. of Dijon mustard

½ Cup of raspberries

1/3 Cup of extra-virgin olive oil

Directions:

Place all the ingredients together except the oil into a blender, according to the ordered list. Cover and blend for 10 seconds by slowly increasing the speed. After 10 seconds, reduce the speed and gradually add the oil into the mixture. Keep the speed at a steady pace until all of the oil has been poured in. Blend until emulsified.

Store in a mason jar, then refrigerate for up to 5 days. Serve with your favorite vegetables or fruit salad.

Nutrition:

Calories: 151 kcal

Protein: 2.22g

Fat: 9.47g

Carbohydrates: 14.65g

256.   Creamy Homemade Greek Dressing

Preparation Time: 10 Minutes
Cooking Time: 0 Minutes
Servings: 2-4
Ingredients:
1/4 Cup of white wine vinegar
2 Tbsp. of lemon or lime juice
1/3 Cup of extra-virgin olive oil
½ Cup of high-quality mayonnaise, without preservatives
2 Cloves of garlic, minced
½ Tsp. dried basil
½ Tsp. dried oregano
½ Tsp. parsley
½ Tsp. thyme
2 Tsp. of honey
¼ Cup non-dairy milk (e.g., almond, rice milk)
A few tablespoons of water
Some Kosher salt and pepper

Directions:
Place all the ingredients together in a mason jar and shake, cover tightly, and shake well. Refrigerate for a few hours before serving or serve immediately on your favorite vegetables or fruit salad.
Shake well before use. Put in the refrigerator for up to 5 days.
You may add a few tablespoons of water to adjust the consistency as per your preference.

Nutrition:
Calories: 474 kcal
Protein: 2.08g
Fat: 50.1g
Carbohydrates: 5.31g

257.   Creamy Siamese Dressing

Preparation Time: 10 Minutes
Cooking Time: 0 Minutes
Servings: 2-4
Ingredients:
1 Cup of mayonnaise
¼ Cup of non-dairy milk (e.g., almond, rice, soymilk)
¼ Cup of unsweetened peanut sauce
2 Tbsp. rice vinegar
1 Tbsp. of honey or maple syrup
1 Tbsp. freshly chopped cilantro
2 Tbsp. of unsalted peanuts

Directions:
Place all ingredients except the cilantro and peanuts into a blender and blend until smooth and creamy.

Then, add in the cilantro and peanuts and pulse the blender a few times until completely crushed and well combined. Put it in a mason jar and bring it to the refrigerator.
Serve with your favorite garden salad, pasta, or as a dipping sauce.

Nutrition:
Calories: 525 kcal
Protein: 18.14g
Fat: 45.55g
Carbohydrates: 11.01g

258.   Honey Bean Dip

Preparation Time: 5 Minutes
Cooking Time: 0 Minutes
Servings: 3-4
Ingredients:
2 Cherry tomatoes
2 Tablespoons filtered water
1 Tablespoon apple cider vinegar
1 (14-ounce) Can of kidney beans and black beans
2 Garlic cloves
¼ Teaspoon ground cumin
¼ Teaspoon salt
2 Teaspoons raw honey
1 Teaspoon lime juice
Pinch cayenne pepper to taste
Freshly ground black pepper to taste

Directions:
In a blender or food processor, put together the beans, garlic, tomatoes, water, vinegar, honey, lime juice, cumin, salt, cayenne pepper, and black pepper. Blend until it turns smooth. Add the mix to a bowl. Cover and refrigerate to chill. You can refrigerate for up to 5 days.

Nutrition:
Calories: 158
Fat: 1g
Carbohydrates: 33g
Fiber: 8g
Protein: 9g

259.   Homemade Ginger Dressing

Preparation Time: 10 Minutes
Cooking Time: 0 Minutes
Servings: 2-4
Ingredients:
1 Cup of chopped onion
Tbsp. of freshly grated ginger

¼ Cup of chopped celery

½ Cup of chopped carrots

1 Tsp. of freshly minced garlic

2/3 Cup of rice vinegar

¼ Cup of water

2 Tbsp. of ketchup

2 ½ Tbsp. of unsalted, gluten-free soy sauce

¼ Cup of honey or maple syrup

1 Tsp. of kosher salt

½ Tsp. of white pepper

1 Cup of extra-virgin olive oil

Directions:

Place the onion, ginger, celery, carrots, and garlic into a blender. Blend until the mixture is fine but still lumpy from the small vegetable chunks.

Add in the vinegar, water, ketchup, soy sauce, honey or maple syrup, lemon juice, salt, and pepper. Pulse until the ingredients are well combined.

Gradually add the oil while blending until everything is well mixed. The mixture should be runny but still grainy.

Serve with your favorite winter salad.

Nutrition:

Calories: 389 kcal

Protein: 2.71g

Fat: 32.08g

Carbohydrates: 22.14g

260. Cucumber and Dill Sauce

Preparation Time: 10 Minutes

Cooking Time: 0 Minutes

Servings: 2-4

Ingredients:

450g of Greek yogurt

1 Cucumber, peeled and squeezed to remove excess liquid

1 Cup of freshly chopped dill

¼ Cup of lemon juice

1 Tsp. of sea salt

Directions:

In a medium bowl, put together the yogurt, cucumber, and dill, then mix until well combined. Add in the lemon juice and salt to taste.

Cover and refrigerate for about 1-2 hours before serving to keep it fresh. Best served with Mediterranean food, chips, fish, or even bread.

Nutrition:

Calories: 97 kcal

Protein: 13.49g Fat: 2.1g

Carbohydrates: 6.34g

261. Cashew Ginger Dip

Preparation Time: 5 Minutes

Cooking Time: 0 Minutes

Servings: 1

Ingredients:

1 Tablespoon extra-virgin olive oil

2 Teaspoons coconut aminos

1 Cup cashews, soaked in water for 20-25 minutes, and drained

2 Garlic cloves

¼ Cup filtered water

1 Teaspoon lemon juice

½ Teaspoon ground ginger

¼ Teaspoon salt

Pinch cayenne pepper

Directions:

In a blender or food processor, put together the cashews, garlic, water, olive oil, aminos, lemon juice, ginger, salt, and cayenne pepper.

Add the mix to a bowl.

Cover and refrigerate until chilled. You can use store it for 4-5 days in the refrigerator.

Nutrition:

Calories:124 Fat:9g

Carbohydrates 5g

Fiber: 1g Protein:3g

262. Bean Potato Spread

Preparation Time: 25 Minutes

Cooking Time: 0 Minutes

Servings: 7-8

Ingredients:

2 Tablespoons lime juice

1 Tablespoon olive oil

Garlic cloves, minced

1 Cup garbanzo beans, drained and rinsed

Cups cooked sweet potatoes, peeled and chopped

¼ Cup sesame paste

½ Teaspoon cumin, ground

2 Tablespoons water

A pinch of salt

Directions:

In a blender, put all the ingredients together and blend to make a smooth mix.

Transfer to a bowl.

Serve with carrot, celery, or veggie sticks.

Nutrition:

Calories:156 Fat:3g

Carbohydrates 10g

Fiber: 6g

Protein:8g

263. Green Beans

Preparation Time: 5 Minutes
Cooking Time: 13 Minutes
Servings: 4
Ingredients:
1 Pound green beans
¾ Teaspoon garlic powder
¾ Teaspoon ground black pepper
1 ¼ Teaspoon salt
½ Teaspoon paprika
Directions:
Turn on the fryer, insert the basket, grease with olive oil, close the lid, set the fryer at 400 degrees F, and preheat for 5 minutes.

Meanwhile, put the beans in a bowl, sprinkle generously with olive oil, sprinkle with garlic powder, black pepper, salt, and paprika and stir until well coated.

Open the air fryer, add the green beans, close with the lid and cook for 8 minutes until golden and crisp, stirring halfway through the frying process.

When the fryer beeps, open the lid, transfer the green beans to a serving plate and serve.

Nutrition:
Calories: 45
Carbs: 2g
Fat: 11g
Protein: 4g
Fiber: 3g

264. Tomato and Mushroom Sauce

Preparation Time: 10 Minutes
Cooking Time: 0 Minutes
Servings: 2-4
Ingredients:
1 Medium-sized leek, chopped
2 Stalks of celery, chopped
2 Medium-sized carrots, chopped
450g of button mushrooms, diced
680g of unsalted tomato puree
½ Cup of water
2 Tsp. of dried oregano
4 Cloves of garlic, crushed
Tbsp. of coconut milk
Some sea salt, seasoning
Black pepper, seasoning
Directions:
In a large skillet, place a few tablespoons of water and heat over medium heat. Once it sizzles, add in the mushrooms and Sautee for about 5 minutes, and stir occasionally.

Next, add in the leek, carrots, and celery. Stir well and cook for about 5 minutes or until the vegetables are tender. Add more water if needed.

Stir in the tomato puree with ½ cup of water and dried oregano. Bring to a boil and then reduce the heat to let it simmer for about 15 minutes.

Take off from heat and mix in the garlic, coconut milk, and salt and pepper to taste.

Put in an airtight container, then store for up to 4 days in the refrigerator or freezer for up to 1 month. Serve with your favorite pasta.

Nutrition:
Calories: 467 kcal
Protein: 16.91g
Fat: 3.81g
Carbohydrates: 109.68g

265. Kale Slaw and Strawberry Salad + Poppy Seeds Dressing

Preparation Time: 10 Minutes
Cooking Time: 20 Minutes
Servings: 2
Ingredients:
Ounces chicken breast sliced and baked
1 Cup Kale chopped
1 Cup Slaw mix (cabbage, broccoli slaw, carrots mixed)
1/4 Cup Slivered almonds
1 Cup Strawberries, sliced
For the dressing:
1 tablespoon Light mayonnaise;
Dijon mustard
1 tablespoon Olive oil
1 tablespoon Apple cider vinegar
½ teaspoon Lemon juice
1 tablespoon of honey
1/4 teaspoon Onion powder
1/4 teaspoon Garlic powder
Poppy seeds
Directions:
Whisk the dressing ingredients together until well mixed, then leave to cool in the fridge.

Slice the chicken breasts.

Divide 2 bowls of spinach, slaw, and strawberries.

Cover with a sliced breast of chicken (4 oz. each), then scatter with almonds.

Divide the dressing between the two bowls and drizzle.

Nutrition:

Calories: 340 Cal

Fats: 13.6g

Saturated Fat: 6.2g

266. Air Fryer Lemon Pepper Shrimp

Difficulty: Average

Preparation Time: 6 minutes

Cooking Time: 11 minutes

Servings: 2

Ingredients:

1 ½ Cup peeled raw shrimps, deveined (1 lean)

½ Tablespoon Olive oil: (1/4 condiment)

Garlic powder: ¼ Tsp. (1/8 condiment)

Lemon pepper: 1 Tsp. (1/4 condiment)

Paprika: ¼ Tsp. (1/8 condiment)

Juice of one lemon (1/4 condiment)

Directions:

Let the air fryer preheat to 400°F

In a bowl, mix lemon pepper, olive oil, paprika, garlic powder, and lemon juice; mix well. Add shrimps and coat well

Add shrimps in the air fryer, cook for 6 or 8 minutes and top with lemon slices and serve

Nutrition:

Calories: 237

Fat: 6g

Protein: 36g

267. Healthy & Tasty Green Beans

Difficulty: Easy

Preparation Time: 10 Minutes

Cooking Time: 10 Minutes

Servings: 2

Ingredients:

2 Cups green beans (½ green)

1/8 Tsp. ground allspice (1/8 condiment)

1/4 Tsp. ground cinnamon (1/8 condiment)

½ Tsp. dried oregano (1/4green)

2 Tbsp. olive oil (1/8 condiment)

1/4 Tsp. ground coriander (1/8 condiment)

1/4 Tsp. ground cumin (1/8 condiment)

1/8 Tsp. cayenne pepper (1/8 condiment)

½ Tsp. salt (1/8 condiment)

Directions:

Add all ingredients into the bowl and toss well.

Add green beans into the air fryer basket and cook at 370°F for 10 minutes. Shake basket halfway through Serve and enjoy.

Nutrition

Calories: 158

Fat: 14g

Protein: 2.1g

268. Cheesy Brussels sprouts

Difficulty: Easy

Preparation Time: 10 Minutes

Cooking Time: 12 Minutes

Servings: 4

Ingredients:

1 lb. Brussels sprouts cut stems and halved (½ green)

1/4 Cup parmesan cheese (½ healthy fat)

1 Tbsp. olive oil (1/4 condiment)

1/4 Tsp. garlic powder (1/4 condiment)

Pepper (1/8 condiment)

Salt (1/8 condiment)

Directions:

Preheat the air fryer to 350°F.

Toss Brussels sprouts, oil, garlic powder, pepper, and salt into the bowl.

Situate Brussels sprouts into the air fryer basket and cook for 12 minutes.

Top with cheese and serve.

Nutrition

Calories: 132 Fat: 7g Protein: 7g

269. Easy Shrimp PO' Boy

Difficulty: Easy

Preparation Time: 19 Minutes

Cooking Time: 9 Minutes

Servings: 4

Ingredients:

2 Cups shredded Iceberg lettuce (1green)

4 Cups deveined shrimps (2 lean)

1/4 Cup buttermilk (1/4 healthy fat)

½ Cup Fish Fry Coating (1/4 condiment)

1 Teaspoon Creole Seasoning (1/8 condiment)

Eight slices of tomato (½ green)

Remoulade Sauce:

½ Tsp. Creole Seasoning (1/8 condiment)

½ Cup Mayo (reduced-fat) (½ healthy fat)

½ Lemon's juice (1/8 condiment)

1 Tsp. Dijon mustard (1/8 condiment)

1 Tsp. Worcestershire (1/8 condiment)

1 Tsp. Minced garlic (1/8 condiment)
1 Green onion chopped (1/4 condiment)
1 Tsp. Hot sauce

Directions:

Remoulade Sauce:

Mix all ingredients in a bowl. Chill in Refrigerator.

Shrimps:

In a zip lock bag, add buttermilk and Creole seasoning with shrimp and mix well; marinate for half an hour.

With cooking oil, spray the air fryer basket. Place the shrimp in the air fryer basket.

Spray the shrimp with olive oil.

Cook at 400°F for five minutes. Flip the shrimps over, and cook for another five minutes.

Add the remolded sauce to whole-wheat bread. Then add tomato slices and lettuce on top, then the shrimp. Enjoy

Nutrition:

Calories: 247
Fat: 19.3g
Protein: 24.7g

270. Air Fryer Garlic-Lime Shrimp Kebabs

Difficulty: Easy
Preparation Time: 5 Minutes
Cooking Time: 19 Minutes
Servings: 2
Ingredients:

1 Lime (1/4 condiment)
1 Cup raw shrimp (1 lean)
Salt: 1/8 teaspoon (1/4 condiment)
1 Clove of garlic (1/4 condiment)
Freshly ground black pepper (1/4 condiment)

Directions:

In water, let wooden skewers soak for 20 minutes.

Let the Air fryer preheat to 350°F.

In a bowl, mix shrimp, minced garlic, lime juice, kosher salt, and pepper

Add shrimp on skewers.

Place skewers in the air fryer, and cook for 8 minutes. Turn halfway over.

Top with cilantro and your favorite dip.

Nutrition:

Calories: 76
Protein: 13g
Fat: 9g

271. Quick & Easy Air Fryer Salmon

Difficulty: Easy
Preparation Time: 6 Minutes
Cooking Time: 13 Minutes
Servings: 4
Ingredients:

2 Teaspoons Lemon pepper seasoning (1/4 condiment)
4 Cups Salmon (2 leans)
1 Tablespoon Olive oil (1/4 condiment)
2 Teaspoons Seafood seasoning (1/4 condiment)
Half lemon's juice (1/4 condiment)
1 Teaspoon Garlic powder (1/8 condiment)
Kosher salt to taste (1/8 condiment)

Directions:

In a bowl, add one tablespoon of olive oil and half lemon juice.

Pour this mixture over salmon and rub. Leave the skin on the salmon. It will come off when cooked.

Rub the salmon with kosher salt and spices.

Put parchment paper in the air fryer basket. Put the salmon in the air fryer.

Cook at 360°F for ten minutes. Cook until inner salmon temperature reaches 140°F.

Let the salmon rest five minutes before serving.

Serve with salad greens and lemon wedges.

Nutrition:

Calories:132
Fat: 7.4g
Protein: 22g

272. Healthy Air Fryer Tuna Patties

Difficulty: Easy
Preparation Time: 15 Minutes
Cooking Time: 11 Minutes
Servings: 10
Ingredients:

½ Cup Whole wheat breadcrumbs (1/4 healthy fat)
4 Cups Fresh tuna, diced (2 leans)
Lemon zest (1/4 condiment)
1 Tablespoon Lemon juice (1/4 condiment)
1 Egg (1/4 healthy fat)
3 Tablespoons Grated parmesan cheese (1/4 healthy fat)
1 Chopped celery stalk (1green)
½ Teaspoon Garlic powder (1/4 condiment)
½ Teaspoon dried herbs (1/4green)
Salt to taste (1/8 condiment)

Freshly ground black pepper (1/8 condiment)

Directions:

In a bowl, add lemon zest, bread crumbs, salt, pepper, celery, eggs, dried herbs, lemon juice, garlic powder, parmesan cheese, and onion. Mix everything. Then add in tuna gently. Shape into patties; if the mixture is too loose, cool in the refrigerator.

Add air fryer baking paper to the air fryer basket. Spray the baking paper with cooking spray.

Spray the patties with oil.

Cook for ten minutes at 360°F. Turn the patties halfway over.

Serve with lemon slices and microgreens.

Nutrition:

Calories: 214

Fat: 15g

Protein: 22g

273. Air Fryer Crispy Fish Sandwich

Difficulty: Easy

Preparation Time: 11 Minutes

Cooking Time: 12 Minutes

Servings: 2

Ingredients:

2 Cod fillets (1 lean)

2 Tablespoons All-purpose flour (1/4 condiment)

1/4 Teaspoon Pepper (1/8 condiment)

1 Tablespoon Lemon juice (1/4 condiment)

1/4 Teaspoon Salt (1/8 condiment)

½ Teaspoon Garlic powder (1/8 condiment)

1 Egg (½ healthy fat)

½ Tablespoon mayo (1/4 healthy fat)

½ Cup Whole wheat bread crumbs (½ healthy fat)

Directions:

In a bowl, add salt, flour, pepper, and garlic powder.

In a separate bowl, add lemon juice, mayo, and egg.

In another bowl, add the breadcrumbs.

Coat the fish in flour, then in egg, then in breadcrumbs.

With cooking oil, spray the basket and put the fish in the basket. Also, spray the fish with cooking oil.

Cook at 400°F for ten minutes. This fish is soft, be careful when you flip it.

Nutrition:

Calories: 218

Fat: 12g

Protein: 22g

274. Garlic Cauliflower Florets

Difficulty: Easy

Preparation Time: 10 Minutes

Cooking Time: 20 minutes

Servings: 4

Ingredients:

4 Cups cauliflower florets (½ green)

½ Tsp. cumin powder (1/8 condiment)

½ Tsp. coriander powder (1/8 condiment)

5 Garlic cloves, chopped (1/8 condiment)

4 tablespoons olive oil (1/8 condiment)

½ Tsp. salt (1/8 condiment)

Directions:

Add all ingredients into the bowl and toss well.

Add cauliflower florets into the air fryer basket and cook at 400 F for 20 minutes. Shake halfway through. Serve and enjoy.

Nutrition:

Calories: 153 Fat: 14g

Protein: 2.3g

275. Breaded Air Fried Shrimp With Bang-Bang Sauce

Difficulty: Difficult

Preparation Time: 9 Minutes

Cooking Time: 22 Minutes

Servings: 4

Ingredients:

3/4 Cup Whole wheat bread crumbs (½ healthy fat)

4 Cups Raw shrimp deveined, peeled (2 leans)

½ Cup Flour (1/8 condiment)

1 Tsp. Paprika (1/8 condiment)

Chicken Seasoning, to taste (1/8 condiment)

2 Tbsp. of one egg white (½ healthy fat)

Kosher salt and pepper to taste (1/8 condiment)

Bang-Bang Sauce:

1/4 Cup sweet chili sauce (1/8 condiment)

1/3 Cup plain Greek yogurt (1/3 healthy fat)

2 Tbsp. Sriracha (1/8 condiment)

Directions:

Let the Air Fryer preheat to 400 degrees.

Add the seasonings to shrimp and coat well.

In three separate bowls, add flour, bread crumbs, and egg whites.

First, coat the shrimps in flour, dab lightly in egg whites, then in the bread crumbs.

With cooking oil, spray the shrimps.

Place the shrimps in an air fryer, cook for four minutes, turn the shrimps over, and cook for another four minutes. Serve with micro green and bang-bang sauce.

Bang-Bang Sauce:
Incorporate all the ingredients and serve.
Nutrition:
Calories: 229
Fat: 10g
Protein: 22g

276.   Delicious Ratatouille

Difficulty: Difficult
Preparation Time: 10 Minutes
Cooking Time: 15 Minutes
Servings: 6
Ingredients:
1 Eggplant, diced (½ green)
3 Garlic cloves, chopped (1/4 condiment)
1 Onion, diced (1/4 condiment)
3 Tomatoes, diced (½ healthy fat)
2 Bell peppers, diced (½ green)
1 Tbsp. vinegar (1/4 condiment)
1 ½ Tbsp. olive oil (1/4 condiment)
2 Tbsp. herb de Provence (½ green)
Pepper (1/8 condiment)
Salt (1/8 condiment)
Directions:
Preheat the air fryer to 400°F.
Add all ingredients into the bowl and toss well.
Add the vegetable mixture into the air fryer basket and cook for 15 minutes. Stir halfway through.
Serve and enjoy.
Nutrition:
Calories: 83
Fat: 4g
Protein: 2g

277.   Simple Green Beans

Difficulty: Easy
Preparation Time: 10 Minutes
Cooking Time: 10 Minutes
Servings: 4
Ingredients:
2 Cups green beans (1green)
1 Tsp. olive oil (½ condiment)
Pepper (1/4 condiment)
Salt (1/4 condiment)
Directions:
In a bowl, toss green beans with oil. Season with pepper and salt.
Transfer green beans into the air fryer basket and cook at 390°F for 10 minutes.
Serve and enjoy.

Nutrition:
Calories: 27
Fat: 1.2g
Protein: 1g

278.   Air Fryer Tofu

Difficulty: Easy
Preparation Time: 10 Minutes
Cooking Time: 15 Minutes
Servings: 4
Ingredients:
15 oz. Extra-firm tofu, cut into bite-sized pieces (1 healthy fat)
1 Tbsp. olive oil (1/4 condiment)
2 Tbsp. soy sauce (1/4 condiment)
1 Garlic clove, minced (1/4 condiment)
Pepper (1/8 condiment)
Salt (1/8 condiment)

Directions:
Add tofu, garlic, oil, soy sauce, pepper, and salt in a bowl and toss well. Set aside for 15 minutes.
Add tofu pieces into the air fryer basket and cook at 370°F for 15 minutes.
Serve and enjoy.
Nutrition:
Calories: 115
Fat: 8g
Protein: 9.8g

279.   Healthy Zucchini Patties

Difficulty: Easy
Preparation Time: 10 Minutes
Cooking Time: 30 Minutes
Servings: 6
Ingredients:
1 Cup zucchini, shredded and squeeze out all liquid (½ green)
1 Egg, lightly beaten (1/4 healthy fat)
1/4 Tsp. red pepper flakes (1/4 condiment)
1/4 Cup parmesan cheese, grated (1/4 healthy fat)
½ Tbsp. Dijon mustard (1/4 condiment)
½ Tbsp. mayonnaise (1/4 healthy fat)
½ Cup breadcrumbs (½ healthy fat)
Pepper (1/8 condiment)
Salt (1/8 condiment)
Directions:
Mix all ingredients into the bowl until well combined.

Make patties from the mixture and place them into the basket and cook at 375°F for 15 minutes.

Turn patties and cook for 15 minutes more.

Serve and enjoy.

Nutrition:

Calories: 80

Fat: 3g

Protein: 4g

280.   Healthy Asparagus Spears

Difficulty: Easy

Preparation Time: 10 Minutes

Cooking Time: 15 Minutes

Servings: 4

Ingredients:

35 Asparagus spears, cut the ends (2green)

½ Tsp. garlic powder (1/4 condiment)

1 Tbsp. olive oil (1/4 condiment)

Pepper (1/8 condiment)

Salt (1/8 condiment)

¼ Tsp. onion powder (1/4 condiment)

Directions:

Add asparagus into the large bowl. Drizzle with oil. Sprinkle with onion powder, garlic powder, pepper, and salt. Toss well.

Arrange asparagus into the air fryer basket and cook at 375°F for 15 minutes.

Serve and enjoy.

Nutrition:

Calories: 75

Fat: 4g

Protein: 4g

281.   Spicy Brussels Sprouts

Difficulty: Easy

Preparation Time: 10 Minutes

Cooking Time: 14 Minutes

Servings: 2

Ingredients:

½ lb. Brussels sprouts, trimmed and halved (1 lean)

½ Tsp. chili powder (1/4 condiment)

1/4 Tsp. cayenne (1/4 condiment)

½ Tbsp. olive oil (1/4 condiment)

1/4 Tsp. smoked paprika (1/4 condiment)

Directions:

Mix all ingredients into the large bowl and toss well.

Add Brussels sprouts into the air fryer basket and cook at 370°F for 14 minutes.

Serve and enjoy.

Nutrition:

Calories: 82

Fat: 4g

Protein: 4g

282.   Asian Green Beans

Difficulty: Average

Preparation Time: 10 Minutes

Cooking Time: 10 Minutes

Servings: 2

Ingredients:

oz. Green beans (1green)

1 Tbsp. tamari (½ condiment)

1 Tsp. sesame oil (½ condiment)

Directions:

Mix all ingredients into the big bowl and toss well.

Add green beans into the air fryer basket and cook at 400°F for 10 minutes.

Serve and enjoy.

Nutrition:

Calories: 60 Fat: 2g

Protein: 3g

283.   Cheese Broccoli Fritters

Difficulty: Average

Preparation Time: 10 Minutes

Cooking Time: 30 Minutes

Servings: 4

Ingredients:

2 Eggs, lightly beaten (½ healthy fat)

3 Cups broccoli florets, cook & mashed (1 lean)

2 Cups cheddar cheese (½ healthy fat)

1/4 Cup almond flour (1/4 condiment)

2 Garlic cloves, minced (1/4 condiment)

Pepper (1/4 condiment)

Salt (1/4 condiment)

Directions:

Mix all ingredients into the bowl.

Make patties from the mixture and place them into the basket and cook at 350°F for 15 minutes.

Turn patties and cook for 15 minutes more.

Serve and enjoy.

Nutrition:

Calories: 285

Fat: 21g

Protein: 18g

284. Air Fryer Bell Peppers

Difficulty: Easy
Preparation Time: 10 Minutes
Cooking Time: 8 Minutes
Servings: 3
Ingredients:
¼ Tsp. onion powder (1/4 condiment)
3 Cups bell peppers, cut into pieces (1green)
1 Tsp. olive oil (½ condiment)
1/4 Tsp. garlic powder (1/4 condiment)
Directions:
Mix all ingredients into the large bowl and toss well.
Transfer bell peppers into the air fryer basket, then cook them at 360°F for 8 minutes. Stir halfway through.
Serve and enjoy.
Nutrition:
Calories: 52
Fat: 2g
Protein: 1.2g

285. Air Fried Tasty Eggplant

Difficulty: Easy
Preparation Time: 10 Minutes
Cooking Time: 12 Minutes
Servings: 2
Ingredients:
1 Eggplant, cut into cubes (1green)
1/4 Tsp. oregano (1/4green)
1 Tbsp. olive oil (½ condiment)
½ Tsp. garlic powder (1/4 condiment)
1/4 Tsp. chili powder (1/4 condiment)
Directions:
Incorporate all ingredients into the huge bowl and toss well.
Transfer into the air fryer basket and cook at 390°F for 12 minutes. Stir halfway through.
Serve and enjoy.
Nutrition
Calories: 120
Fat: 7g
Protein: 2g

286. Spicy Asian Brussels sprouts

Difficulty: Average
Preparation Time: 10 Minutes
Cooking Time: 15 Minutes
Servings: 4
Ingredients:
1 lb. Brussels sprouts, cut in half (1green)

1 Tbsp. gochujang (½ condiment)
1 ½ Tbsp. olive oil (1/4 condiment)
½ Tsp. salt (1/4 condiment)
Directions:
In a bowl, mix olive oil, gochujang, and salt.
Add Brussels sprouts into the bowl and toss until well coated.
Add Brussels sprouts into the air fryer basket and cook at 360°F for 15 minutes.
Serve and enjoy.
Nutrition
Calories: 94
Fat: 5g
Protein: 4g

287. Healthy Mushrooms

Difficulty: Easy
Preparation Time: 10 Minutes
Cooking Time: 12 Minutes
Servings: 2
Ingredients:
oz. Mushrooms, clean and cut into quarters (2 healthy fats)
1 Tbsp. fresh parsley, chopped (½ green)
1 Tsp. soy sauce (1/4 condiment)
½ Tsp. garlic powder (1/4 condiment)
1 Tbsp. olive oil (1/4 condiment)
Pepper (1/8 condiment)
Salt (1/8 condiment)
Directions:
Add mushrooms and remaining ingredients into the bowl and toss well.
Add the mushrooms into the air fryer basket and cook at 380°F for 12 minutes. Stir halfway through.
Serve and enjoy.
Nutrition
Calories: 90
Fat: 7g
Protein: 4g

288. Cheese Stuff Peppers

Difficulty: Average
Preparation Time: 10 Minutes
Cooking Time: 8 Minutes
Servings: 4
Ingredients:
Jalapeno peppers, halved, remove seeds and stem (4 leans)
½ Cup cheddar cheese (1/4 healthy fat)

½ Cup Monterey jack cheese, shredded (1/4 healthy fat)

oz. Cream cheese softened (½ healthy fat)

Directions:

In a bowl, mix together cheddar, Monterey jack cheese, and cream cheese.

Stuff cheese mixture into jalapeno halved.

Place the jalapeno peppers into the air fryer basket and cook at 370°F for 8 minutes.

Serve and enjoy.

Nutrition

Calories: 365

Fat: 33g

Protein: 13.2g

289. Cheesy Broccoli Cauliflower

Difficulty: Easy

Preparation Time: 10 Minutes

Cooking Time: 20 Minutes

Servings: 6

Ingredients:

4 Cups cauliflower florets (1green)

4 Cups broccoli florets (1green)

2/3 Cups parmesan cheese, shredded (1 healthy fat)

5 Garlic cloves, minced (½ condiment)

1/3 Cup olive oil (1/4 condiment)

Pepper (1/8 condiment)

Salt (1/8 condiment)

Directions:

Add half cheese, broccoli, cauliflower, garlic, oil, pepper, and salt into the bowl and toss well.

Add broccoli and cauliflower to the air fryer basket and cook at 370°F for 20 minutes.

Add remaining cheese. Toss well.

Serve and enjoy.

Nutrition

Calories: 165

Fat: 13.6g

Protein: 6.4g

290. Air Fryer Broccoli & Brussels Sprouts

Difficulty: Average

Preparation Time: 10 Minutes

Cooking Time: 30 Minutes

Servings: 6

Ingredients:

1 lb. Brussels sprouts, cut ends (1green)

1 lb. Broccoli, cut into florets (1green)

1 Tsp. paprika (1/4 condiment)

1 Tsp. garlic powder (1/4 condiment)

½ Tsp. pepper (1/4 condiment)

3 Tbsp. olive oil (1 healthy fat)

3/4 Tsp. salt (1/4 condiment)

Directions:

Add all ingredients into the bowl and toss well.

Add the vegetable mixture into the air fryer basket and cook at 370°F for 30 minutes.

Serve and enjoy.

Nutrition

Calories: 125

Fat: 7.6g

Protein: 5g

291. Spicy Asparagus Spears

Difficulty: Easy

Preparation Time: 10 Minutes

Cooking Time: 15 Minutes

Servings: 4

Ingredients:

35 Asparagus spears, cut the ends (2green)

½ Tsp. chili powder (1/4 condiment)

1/4 Tsp. paprika (1/4 condiment)

1 Tbsp. olive oil (1/4 condiment)

Pepper (1/8 condiment)

Salt (1/8 condiment)

Directions:

Add asparagus into the large bowl. Drizzle with oil. Sprinkle with paprika, chili powder, pepper, and salt. Toss well. Add asparagus into the air fryer basket and cook at 400°F for 15 minutes.

Serve and enjoy.

Nutrition

Calories: 75 Fat: 3.8g Protein: 4.7g

292. Almond Flour Battered 'n Crisped Onion Rings

Difficulty: Average

Preparation Time: 10 Minutes

Cooking Time: 15 Minutes

Servings: 3

Ingredients:

½ Cup almond flour (1/4 healthy fat)

¾ Cup coconut milk (1/4 healthy fat)

1 Big white onion, sliced into rings (1green)

1 Egg, beaten (1/4 healthy fat)

1 Tablespoon baking powder (1/4 condiment)

1 Tablespoon smoked paprika (1/4 condiment)

Salt and pepper to taste (1/8 condiment)

Directions:

Preheat the air fryer for 5 minutes.

In a mixing bowl, mix the almond flour, baking powder, smoked paprika, salt, and pepper.

In another bowl, combine the eggs and coconut milk.

Soak the onion slices into the egg mixture.

Dredge the onion slices in the almond flour mixture.

Place in the air fryer basket.

Close and cook for 15 minutes at 325°F.

Halfway through the cooking time, shake the fryer basket for even cooking.

Nutrition:

Calories: 217 Protein: 5.3g Fat: 18g

293. Mediterranean-Style Eggs With Spinach

Difficulty: Easy

Preparation Time: 3 Minutes

Cooking Time: 12 Minutes

Servings: 2

Ingredients:

2 Tablespoons olive oil, melted (1/4 condiment)

4 Eggs, whisked (1 healthy fat)

5 Ounces fresh spinach, chopped (1green)

1 Medium-sized tomato, chopped (1green)

1 Teaspoon fresh lemon juice (1/4 condiment)

½ Teaspoon coarse salt (1/8 condiment)

½ Teaspoon ground black pepper (1/8 condiment)

½ Cup of fresh basil, roughly chopped (1/4green)

Directions:

Add the olive oil to an Air Fryer baking pan. Make sure to tilt the pan to spread the oil evenly.

Simply combine the remaining ingredients, except for the basil leaves; whisk well until everything is well incorporated.

Cook in the preheated oven for 8 to 12 minutes at 280 degrees F. Garnish with fresh basil leaves. Serve.

Nutrition:

Calories: 274 Fat: 23g Protein: 14g

294. Tomato Bites With Creamy Parmesan Sauce

Difficulty: Easy

Preparation Time: 7 Minutes

Cooking Time: 13 Minutes

Servings: 4

Ingredients:

For the Sauce:

½ Cup Parmigiano-Reggiano cheese, grated (1/4 healthy fat)

4 Tablespoons pecans, chopped (½ healthy fat)

1 Teaspoon garlic puree (1/8 condiment)

½ Teaspoon fine sea salt (1/8 condiment)

1/3 Cup extra-virgin olive oil (1/8 condiment)

For the Tomato Bites:

2 Large-sized Roma tomatoes, cut into thin slices and pat them dry (1green)

Ounces Halloumi cheese, cut into thin slices (1 healthy fat)

1 Teaspoon dried basil (½ green)

1/4 Teaspoon red pepper flakes, crushed (1/8 condiment)

1/8 Teaspoon sea salt (1/8 condiment)

Directions:

Start by preheating your Air Fryer to 385 degrees F. Make the sauce by mixing all ingredients, except the extra-virgin olive oil, in your food processor.

While the machine is running, slowly and gradually pour in the olive oil; puree until everything is well blended.

Now, spread one teaspoon of the sauce over the top of each tomato slice. Place a slice of Halloumi cheese on each tomato slice. Top with onion slices. Sprinkle with basil, red pepper, and sea salt.

Transfer the assembled bites to the Air Fryer. Spray with non-stick cooking spray and cook for about 13 minutes.

Arrange these bites on a nice serving platter, garnish with the remaining sauce, and serve at room temperature. Bon appétit!

Nutrition:

Calories: 428

Fat: 38g

Protein: 18g

295. Spicy Zesty Broccoli With Tomato Sauce

Difficulty: Average

Preparation Time: 5 Minutes

Cooking Time: 15 Minutes

Servings: 6

Ingredients:

For the Broccoli Bites:

1 Medium-sized head broccoli, broken into florets (1green)

½ Teaspoon lemon zest, freshly grated (1/4 condiment)

1/3 Teaspoon fine sea salt (1/8 condiment)

½ Teaspoon hot paprika (1/8 condiment)

1 Teaspoon shallot powder (1/8 condiment)

1 Teaspoon porcini powder (1/8 condiment)

½ Teaspoon granulated garlic (1/8 condiment)

1/3 Teaspoon celery seeds (1/4 healthy fat)

1 ½ Tablespoons olive oil (1/8 condiment)

For the Hot Sauce:

½ Cup tomato sauce (½ healthy fat)

1 Tablespoon balsamic vinegar (1/8 condiment)

½ Teaspoon ground allspice (1/8 condiment)

Directions:

Toss all the ingredients for the broccoli bites in a mixing bowl, covering the broccoli florets on all sides. Cook them in the preheated Air Fryer at 360 degrees for 13 to 15 minutes. In the meantime, mix all ingredients for the hot sauce.

Pause your Air Fryer, mix the broccoli with the prepared sauce and cook for a further 3 minutes. Bon appétit!

Nutrition:

Calories: 70

Fat: 4g

Protein: 2g

296.   Cheese Stuffed Mushrooms With Horseradish Sauce

Difficulty: Average

Preparation Time: 3 Minutes

Cooking Time: 12 Minutes

Servings: 5

Ingredients:

½ Cup parmesan cheese, grated (1/4 healthy fat)

2 Cloves garlic, pressed (1/4 condiment)

2 Tablespoons fresh coriander, chopped (1/4green)

1/3 Teaspoon kosher salt (1/8 condiment)

½ Teaspoon crushed red pepper flakes (1/8 condiment)

1 ½ Tablespoon olive oil (1/4 condiment)

20 Medium-sized mushrooms, cut off the stems (1 healthy fat)

½ Cup Gorgonzola cheese, grated (½ healthy fat)

1/4 Cup low-fat mayonnaise (1/4 healthy fat)

1 Teaspoon prepared horseradish, well-drained (1/4green)

1 Tablespoon fresh parsley, finely chopped (1/4green)

Directions:

Mix the parmesan cheese together with the garlic, coriander, salt, red pepper, and olive oil; mix to combine well.

Stuff the mushroom caps with the cheese filling. Top them with grated Gorgonzola.

Place the mushrooms in the Air Fryer grill pan and slide them into the machine. Grill them at 380 degrees F for 8 to 12 minutes or until the stuffing is warmed through.

Meanwhile, prepare the horseradish sauce by mixing mayonnaise, horseradish, and parsley. Serve the horseradish sauce with warm fried mushrooms. Enjoy!

Nutrition:

Calories: 180 Fat: 13.2g

Protein: 9g

297.   Broccoli With Herbs and Cheese

Difficulty: Average

Preparation Time: 8 Minutes

Cooking Time: 17 Minutes

Servings: 4

Ingredients:

1/3 Cup grated yellow cheese (½ healthy fat)

1 Large-sized head broccoli, stemmed and cut small florets (1green)

2 ½ Tablespoons canola oil (1/8 condiment)

2 Teaspoons dried rosemary (1/4green)

2 Teaspoons dried basil (1/4green)

Salt and ground black pepper to taste (1/8 condiment)

Directions:

Bring a medium pan filled with lightly salted water to a boil. Then, boil the broccoli florets for about 3 minutes.

Then, drain the broccoli florets well; toss them with canola oil, rosemary, basil, salt, and black pepper.

Set your oven to 390 degrees F; arrange the seasoned broccoli in the cooking basket; set the timer for 17 minutes. Toss the broccoli halfway through the cooking process.

Serve warm topped with grated cheese, and enjoy!

Nutrition:

Calories: 111 Fat: 2.1g Protein: 8.9g

298.   Family Favorite Stuffed Mushrooms

Difficulty: Easy

Preparation Time: 4 Minutes

Cooking Time: 12 Minutes

Servings: 2

Ingredients:

2 Teaspoons cumin powder (1/4 condiment)

4 Garlic cloves, peeled and minced (1/4 condiment)

18 Medium-sized white mushrooms (2 healthy fats)
Fine sea salt and freshly ground black pepper to taste (1/8 condiment)
A pinch ground allspice (1/8 condiment)
2 Tablespoons olive oil (1/4 condiment)

Directions:

First, clean the mushrooms; remove the middle stalks from the mushrooms to prepare the "shells." Grab a mixing dish and thoroughly combine the remaining items. Fill the mushrooms with the prepared mixture.

Cook the mushrooms at 345 degrees F heat for 12 minutes. Enjoy!

Nutrition:

Calories: 179

Fat: 15g

Protein: 6g

299. Spanish-Style Eggs With Manchego Cheese

Difficulty: Difficult

Preparation Time: 10 Minutes

Cooking Time: 38 Minutes

Servings: 4

Ingredients:

1/3 Cup grated Manchego cheese (½ healthy fat)
5 Eggs (2 healthy fats)
2 Green garlic stalks, peeled and finely minced (1green)
1 ½ Cups white mushrooms, chopped (1 healthy fat)
1 Teaspoon dried basil (1/4green)
1 ½ Tablespoon olive oil (½ condiment)
3/4 Teaspoons dried oregano (1/4green)
½ Teaspoon dried parsley flakes or one tablespoon fresh flat-leaf Italian parsley (1/4green)
1 Teaspoon porcini powder (1/8 condiment)
Table salt and freshly ground black pepper to taste (1/8 condiment)

Directions:

Start by preheating your Air Fryer to 350 degrees F. Add the oil, mushrooms, and green garlic to the Air Fryer baking dish. Bake the mixture for 6 minutes or until tender.

Meanwhile, crack the eggs into a mixing bowl; beat the eggs until they're well whisked. Next, add the seasonings and mix again. Pause your Air Fryer and take the baking dish out of the basket.

Pour the whisked egg mixture into the baking dish with sautéed mixture. Top with the grated Manchego cheese.

Bake for about 32 minutes at 320 degrees F or until your frittata is set. Serve warm. Bon appétit!

Nutrition:

Calories: 153

Fat: 12g

Protein: 9g

300. Famous Fried Pickles

Difficulty: Average

Preparation Time: 5 Minutes

Cooking Time: 15 Minutes

Servings: 6

Ingredients:

1/3 Cup milk (½ healthy fat)
1 Teaspoon garlic powder (1/8 condiment)
2 Medium-sized eggs (1 healthy fat)
1 Teaspoon fine sea salt (1/8 condiment)
1/3 Teaspoon chili powder (1/4 condiment)
1/3 Cup all-purpose flour (1/4 healthy fat)
½ Teaspoon shallot powder (1/4 condiment)
2 Jars sweet and sour pickle spears (1 healthy fat)

Directions:

Pat the pickle spears dry with a kitchen towel. Then take two mixing bowls.

Whisk the egg and milk in a bowl. In another bowl, combine all dry ingredients.

Firstly, dip the pickle spears into the dry mix; then coat each pickle with the egg/milk mixture; dredge them in the flour mixture again for additional coating. Air fry battered pickles for 15 minutes at 385 degrees. Enjoy!

Nutrition:

Calories: 58

Fat: 2g

Protein: 3.2g

301. Fried Squash Croquettes

Difficulty: Easy

Preparation Time: 5 Minutes

Cooking Time: 17 Minutes

Servings: 4

Ingredients:

1/3 Cup all-purpose flour (1/4 condiment)
1/3 Teaspoon freshly ground black pepper, or more to taste (1/4 condiment)
1/3 Teaspoon dried sage (1/8 condiment)
4 Cloves garlic, minced (1/4 condiment)
1 ½ Tablespoon olive oil (1/4 condiment)
1/3 Butternut squash, peeled and grated
2 Eggs, well whisked (1 healthy fat)

1 Teaspoon fine sea salt (1/8 condiment)
A pinch of ground allspice (1/8 condiment)
Directions:
Thoroughly combine all ingredients in a mixing bowl. Preheat your Air Fryer to 345 degrees and set the timer for 17 minutes; cook until your fritters are browned; serve right away.
Nutrition:
Calories: 152
Fat: 10g
Protein: 6g

302.   Cauliflower Crust Pizza

Difficulty: Average
Preparation Time: 20 Minutes
Cooking Time: 45 Minutes
Servings: 4
Ingredients:
1 Cauliflower (1green)
¼ Grated parmesan cheese (½ healthy fat)
1 Egg (1/4 healthy fat)
1 Tsp. Italian seasoning (1/8 condiment)
1/4 Tsp. kosher salt (1/8 condiment)
2 Cups of freshly grated mozzarella (1/4 healthy fat)
1/4 Cup of spicy pizza sauce (1/8 condiment)
Basil leaves for garnishing (1/4green)
Directions:
Begin by preheating your oven while using the parchment paper to rim the baking sheet.
Process the cauliflower into a fine powder and then transfer to a bowl before putting it into the microwave.
Leave for about 5-6 minutes to get it soft.
Transfer the microwaved cauliflower to a clean and dry kitchen towel.
Leave it to cool off.
When cold, use the kitchen towel to wrap the cauliflower and then get rid of all the moisture by wringing the towel.
Continue squeezing until the water is gone completely.
Put the cauliflower, Italian seasoning, Parmesan, egg, salt, and mozzarella (1 cup).
Stir very well until well combined.
Transfer the combined mixture to the baking sheet previously prepared, pressing it into a 10-inch round shape.
Bake for 10-15 minutes until it becomes golden in color.

Take the baked crust out of the oven and use the spicy pizza sauce and mozzarella (the leftover 1 cup) to top it.
Bake again for ten more minutes until the cheese melts and looks bubbly.
Garnish using fresh basil leaves. You can also enjoy this with salad.
Nutrition:
Calories: 74
Protein: 6g
Fat: 4g

303.   Tamarind   Glazed   Sweet Potatoes

Difficulty: Easy
Preparation Time: 2 Minutes
Cooking Time: 22 Minutes
Servings: 4
Ingredients:
1/3 Teaspoon white pepper (1/8 condiment)
1 Tablespoon butter, melted (1/4 healthy fat)
½ Teaspoon turmeric powder (1/8 condiment)
5 Garnet sweet potatoes, peeled and diced (2 healthy fat)
A few drops of liquid Stevia (1/8 condiment)
2 Teaspoons tamarind paste (1/4 condiment)
1 ½ Tablespoons fresh lime juice (1/8 condiment)
1 ½ Teaspoon ground allspice (1/8 condiment)
Directions:
In a mixing bowl, toss all ingredients until sweet potatoes are well coated.
Air-fry them at 335 degrees F for 12 minutes.
Pause the Air Fryer and toss again. Increase the temperature to 390 degrees F and cook for an additional 10 minutes. Eat warm.
Nutrition:
Calories: 103
Fat: 9g
Protein: 1.9g

304.   Nicoise Salad

Preparation Time: 10 minutes
Cooking Time: 20 minutes
Servings: 4
Ingredients:
½ cup of pitted Kalamata olives
2 (5 ounces) cans of solid-packed tuna in oil, should be drained
1/3 cup of olive oil
¼ teaspoon of dried thyme

¼ teaspoon of black pepper

¼ teaspoon of salt

1 tablespoon of Dijon mustard

3 tablespoons of white balsamic or white wine vinegar

¾ cup of dry-packed sun-dried tomatoes, should be halved

4 large eggs

1 (12 ounces) package of frozen whole green beans

1 (20 0unce) package of roasted red potatoes

Directions:

Check the package directions on the beans and potatoes to cook them.

Get a saucepan and put the eggs before adding cold water on top of it, place it on the heat to boil. Once boiled, remove it from the heat, cover it, and leave it for about 12 minutes. Next is to drain it and put the eggs inside cold water before peeling. Cut each of the eggs into 2 lengthwise.

Pour tomatoes in boiling water for 30 seconds to soften it. Then drain.

Get a bowl and whisk together thyme, pepper, salt, mustard, and vinegar in a bowl. Add oil gradually until they are well-combined.

Get a platter to arrange the olives, tuna, eggs, tomatoes, beans, and potatoes and drizzle dressing on it.

Nutrition: 598.9 Calories, 31.7g Protein, 45.3g Carbohydrate, 33 g Fat, Sodium: 1039.8mg , Cholesterol: 197.6mg , Sugars: 8g

305.   Zucchini Mint Salad

Preparation Time: 10 minutes, Additional Time: 5 minutes

Cooking Time: 0

Servings: 2

Total Time: 15 minutes

Ingredients:

Ground black pepper and salt to taste

1 tablespoon of chopped fresh mint

1 tablespoon of freshly squeezed lemon juice

1 tablespoon of extra-virgin olive oil

1 small yellow squash, should be cut into ¼ - inch rounds

1 small zucchini, should be cut into ¼ - inch rounds

Directions:

Arrange the yellow squash rounds and zucchini inside a plate and sprinkle all over with salt. Put it aside and wait for about 5 minutes for its water to pull out.

Then drizzle yellow squash and zucchini with lemon juice and olive oil and sprinkle mint over it. Finally, sprinkle with black pepper.

Nutrition: 90.9 Calories, 1.7g Protein, 6.7g Carbohydrate, 7.1 g Fat, Sodium: 8mg , Cholesterol: 0mg , Sugars: 1.2g

306.   Herb Potatoes

Preparation Time: 5 minutes

Cooking Time: 40 minutes

Servings: 5

Ingredients:

2 medium (2-1/4" to 3" dia, raw)s of red potatoes, to be chopped

3 large carrots, should be sliced diagonally

2 small Vidalia onions, should be wedged

¼ teaspoon of ground black pepper

1 teaspoon of dried rosemary, should be crushed

1 teaspoon of garlic salt

1 tablespoon of balsamic vinegar

2 tablespoons of olive oil

Directions:

Get your barbeque on high heat or preheat your oven to 4000F (2000C)

You will need a 9x13 inch baking dish to mix the ground black pepper, rosemary, garlic salt, vinegar, and olive oil. Put the onions, potatoes, and carrots inside the dish and toss all together to have a coat.

Grill or bake, and turn as often as possible until it becomes tender; this should take about 40 minutes.

Nutrition: 152.9 Calories, 2.7g Protein, 23.7g Carbohydrate, 5.7g Fat, Sodium: 385.6mg , Cholesterol: 0mg , Sugars: 6.5g

307.   Fresh Green Bean Salad

Preparation Time: 20 minutes

Cooking Time: 5 minutes

Servings: 8

Ingredients:

Dressing:

Ground pepper and salt to taste

1 tablespoon of vinegar

1 tablespoon of olive oil

Salad:

3 eaches of cucumbers, to be chopped

1 bunch of radishes. To be chopped

2 pounds of fresh green beans, to be trimmed

Directions:

Get a pot, add water and a little salt in it and get it to boil, then add beans in the boiling water and cook until it becomes slightly tender and bright green in about 3-5 minutes. After that, drain the green beans and pour it inside ice water until it becomes cold; then drain it.

Get a large bowl to toss cucumbers, radishes, and green beans together.

Get a small-size bowl and whisk vinegar and olive oil together until they both become an emulsion, then season with pepper and salt. Place the dressing on top of the salad and toss it to have a coat.

Nutrition: 67.6 Calories, 2.8g Protein, 12.3g Carbohydrate, 2 g Fat, Sodium: 13mg , Cholesterol: 0mg , Sugars: 3.5g

308. Roasted Garlic Cauliflower

Preparation Time: 15 minutes
Cooking Time: 25 minutes
Servings: 6
Ingredients:

1 tablespoon of chopped fresh parsley
Black pepper and salt to taste
1/3 cup of grated Parmesan cheese
1 large head of cauliflower, should be separated into florets
3 tablespoons of olive oil
2 tablespoons of minced garlic

Directions:

Let your oven preheat to 450°F (220°C). Get your large casserole dish greased lightly.

Get a resealable bag and put the garlic and olive oil. Then add cauliflower and shake very well to have a mix. Next is to pour the mixture inside the casserole dish and season with pepper and salt to taste.

Let it bake for about 25 minutes and stir occasionally. You should top it with parsley and Parmesan cheese and broil for about 5 minutes till it becomes golden brown.

Nutrition: 118.2 Calories, 4.7g Protein, 8.6g Carbohydrate, 8.2 g Fat, Sodium: 110.9mg , Cholesterol: 3.9mg , Sugars: 3.4g

309. Grilled Green Beans

Preparation Time: 5 minutes
Cooking Time: 10 minutes, Additional Time: 30 minutes
Servings: 4
Total Time: 45 minutes
Ingredients:

1 teaspoon of kosher salt
1 teaspoon of minced garlic
¼ cup of olive oil
1 pound of fresh green beans, should be trimmed

Directions:

Get a bowl and combine salt, garlic, olive oil, and green beans inside it; toss together to have a coat. Then give the green beans about 30 minutes to marinate.

Preheat your grill over medium heat and oil the grate lightly. Then, get a grill pan to lay the green beans.

Next is to put the grill pan on the already preheated grill, then cook and stir the green beans for about 10 minutes or until it becomes lightly charred.

Nutrition: 155.6 Calories, 2.1g Protein, 8.3g Carbohydrate, 13.6 g Fat, Sodium: 487.2mg , Cholesterol: 0mg , Sugars: 1.6g

310. Kale Caesar

Preparation Time: 15 minutes
Cooking Time: 0
Servings: 4
Ingredients:

¼ cup of grated Parmesan cheese
1 cup of croutons
6 cups of kale leaves
Ground black pepper as desired
¼ teaspoon of salt
½ cup of olive oil
½ teaspoon of Dijon mustard
2 cloves of garlic, should be peeled
2 anchovies of anchovy fillets
½ cup of lemon juice

Directions:

Get a blender or food processor with a fitted steel blade and combine mustard, garlic, anchovies, and lemon juice inside. Let it process until they are all thoroughly combined. While the machine is running, gradually pour in the olive oil through the feed tube; you should do it 1 tbsp. at first before increasing it to 2, 3, etc. or as convenient for you. Next is to season with pepper and salt.

Get a cutting board to stack the kale leaves together and cut through the stack in skinny slivers.

Get a bowl and put Parmesan cheese, croutons, and kale and drizzle a quarter of the dressing on it. Toss together and taste it; you may add more dressing if needed, but remember to toss it again after doing that.

Nutrition: 361.5 Calories, 6.8g Protein, 17.6g Carbohydrate, 31.1 g Fat, Sodium: 437.3mg , Cholesterol: 6.1mg , Sugars: 1.2g

311. Rosemary Cauliflower Rolls

Preparation Time: 10 minutes
Cooking Time: 30 minutes
Servings: 3
Ingredients:
1/3 cup of almond flour
4 cups of riced cauliflower
1/3 cup of reduced-fat, shredded mozzarella or cheddar cheese
2 eggs
2 tablespoon of fresh rosemary, finely chopped
½ teaspoon of salt
Directions:
Preheat your oven to 4000F
Combine all the listed ingredients in a medium-sized bowl
Scoop cauliflower mixture into 12 evenly-sized rolls/biscuits onto a lightly-greased and foil-lined baking sheet.
Bake until it turns golden brown, which should be achieved in about 30 minutes.
Note: if you want to have the outside of the rolls/biscuits crisp, then broil for some minutes before serving.
Nutrition: Calories: 254Protein: 24gCarbohydrate: 7gFat: 8 g

Chapter 6:

Dinner Recipes

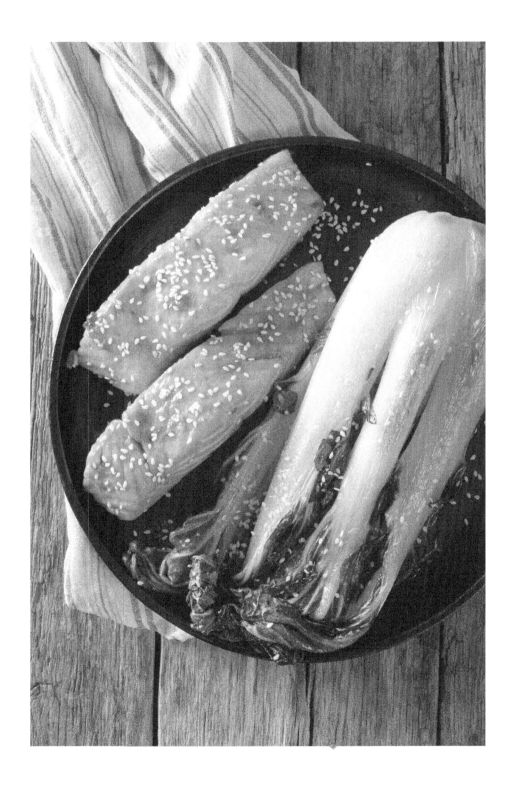

312. October Potato Soup

Prep Time : 8 mins
Cook Time : 20 mins
Servings : 3
Ingredients :
4 minced garlic cloves
2 teaspoon coconut oil
3 diced celery stalks
1 diced onion
2 teaspoon yellow mustard seeds
5 diced Yukon potatoes
cups vegetable broth
1 teaspoon oregano
1 teaspoon paprika
1/2 teaspoon cayenne pepper
1 teaspoon chili powder
Salt and pepper to taste
Directions :
Begin by sautéing the garlic and the mustard seeds together in the oil in a large soup pot.
Next, add the onion and sauté the mixture for another five minutes.
Add the celery, the broth, the potatoes, and all the spices, and continue to stir.
Allow the soup to simmer for thirty minutes without a cover.
Next, Position about three cups of the soup in a blender, and puree the soup until you've reached a smooth consistency. Pour this back into the big soup pot, stir, and serve warm. 7
Nutrition : Calories 200; Carbs: 10g ;Fat: 6g; Protein: 7g

313. Red Quinoa and Black Bean Soup

Prep Time : 6 mins
Cook Time : 40 mins
Servings : 6
Ingredients :
1 1/4 cup red quinoa
4 minced garlic cloves
1/2 tablespoon coconut oil
1 diced jalapeno
3 cups diced onion
2 teaspoon cumin
1 chopped sweet potato
1 teaspoon coriander
1 teaspoon chili powder
5 cups vegetable broth
15 ounces black beans

1/2 teaspoon cayenne pepper
2 cups spinach
Directions :
Begin by bringing the quinoa into a saucepan to boil with two cups of water. Allow the quinoa to simmer for twenty minutes. Next, remove the quinoa from the heat.
To the side, heat the oil, the onion, and the garlic together in a large soup pot.
Add the jalapeno and the sweet potato and sauté for an additional seven minutes.
Next, add all the spices and the broth and bring the soup to a simmer for twenty-five minutes. The potatoes should be soft.
Prior to serving, add the quinoa, the black beans, and the spinach to the mix. Season, and serve warm.
Nutrition : Calories 208; Carbs: 20g ; Fat: 5g; Protein: 17g

314. Tilapia and Broccoli

Prep Time : 5 mins
Cook Time : 14 mins
Servings : 1
Ingredients :
oz. tilapia, frozen is fine
1 T butter
1 T garlic, minced or finely chopped
1 teaspoon of lemon pepper seasoning
1 cup broccoli florets, fresh or frozen, but fresh will be crisper
Directions :
Set the pre-warmed oven for 350 degrees.
Place the fish in an aluminum foil packet.
Arrange the broccoli around the fish to make an attractive arrangement.
Sprinkle the lemon pepper on the fish.
Close the packet and seal, bake for 14 minutes.
Combine the garlic and butter. Set aside.
Remove the packet from the oven and transfer ingredients to a plate. Place the butter on the fish and broccoli. **Nutrition :** Calories 360; Total Fat: 23g ; Protein: 27g; Carbs: 3.2g

315. Chicken Relleno Casserole

Prep Time : 20 mins
Cook Time : 29 mins
Servings : 6
Ingredients :
6 Tortilla Factory low-carb whole wheat tortillas, torn into small pieces

1 ½ cups hand-shredded cheese, Mexican
1 beaten egg
1 cup milk
2 cups cooked chicken, shredded
1 can Ro-tel
½ cup salsa verde
Directions :
Grease an 8 x 8 glass baking dish
Heat oven to 375 degrees
Combine everything together, but reserve ½ cup of the cheese
Bake it for 29 minutes
Take it out of oven and add ½ cup cheese
Broil for about 2 minutes to melt the cheese
Nutrition :
Calories 260
Fat: 15g
Protein: 18g
Carbs: 16g

316. Italian Chicken with Asparagus and Artichoke Hearts

Prep Time : 10 mins
Cook Time : 40 mins
Servings : 1
Ingredients :
1 can long asparagus spears, drained
1 c red peppers, roasted, drained
1 c artichoke hearts, drained
6 oz. of boneless chicken breast, pounded thin or sliced thinly
2 T parmesan cheese
1 T Bisquick
½ teaspoon oregano
½ teaspoon garlic powder
½ cup fresh sliced mushrooms
2 T red wine vinegar
2 T butter
3 T olive oil
Directions :
Place in a small blender container (or bowl) the oregano, garlic powder, vinegar, and 1 T oil.
Place to the side.
Combine the Bisquick and Parmesan cheese. Roll the chicken in the Bisquick and Parmesan mix.
Heat the butter in a skillet.
Brown the chicken on both sides and cook until done, approximately 4 minutes.
Emulsify or quickly whip the wet ingredients you have placed to the side. This is your dressing.

Place the chicken on the plate.
Surround with the vegetables and drizzle them with the dressing.
Nutrition:
Calories 430
Fat: 16g
Protein: 37g
Carbs: 15g

317. Walnut and Date Porridge

Prep Time : 12 mins
Cook Time : 10 mins
Servings : 1
Ingredients :
Strawberries, ½ cup (hulled)
Milk or dairy-free alternative, 200 ml
Buckwheat flakes, ½ cup
Medjool date, 1 (chopped)
Walnut butter, 1 teaspoon, or chopped walnut halves
Directions :
Place the date and the milk in a pan, heat gently before adding the buckwheat flakes. Then cook until the porridge gets to your desired consistency.
Add the walnuts, stir, then top with the strawberries. Serve.
Nutrition :
Calories: 250
Protein: 63 g
Fat: 3 g
Vitamin B

318. Kabobs with Peanut Curry Sauce

Prep Time : 10 mins
Cook Time : 9 mins
Servings : 4
Ingredients :
1 cup Cream
4 teaspoon Curry Powder
1 1/2 teaspoon Cumin
1 1/2 teaspoon Salt
1 T minced garlic
1/3 cup Peanut Butter, sugar-free
2 T Lime Juice
3 T Water
1/2 small Onion, diced
2 T Soy Sauce
1 packet Splenda
oz. boneless, cooked Chicken Breast
oz. pork tenderloin

114

Directions :

Blend together cream, onion, 2 teaspoon. garlic, curry and cumin powder, and salt.

Slice the meats into 1 inch pieces.

Place the cream sauce into a bowl and put in the chicken and tenderloin to marinate. Let rest in sauce for 14 minutes.

Blend peanut butter, water, 1 teaspoon. garlic, lime juice, soy sauce, and Splenda. This is your peanut dipping sauce.

Remove the meats and thread on skewers. Broil or grill 4 minutes per side until meat is done. Serve with dipping sauce.

Nutrition : Calories 525; Fat: 26g ; Protein: 35g; Carbs: 5g

319.   Salmon with Bok-Choy

Prep Time : 10 mins
Cook Time : 9 mins
Servings : 4
Ingredients :

1 c red peppers, roasted, drained
2 cups chopped bok-choy
1 T salted butter
5 oz. salmon steak
1 lemon, sliced very thinly
1/8 teaspoon black pepper
1 T olive oil
2 T sriracha sauce

Directions :

Place oil in skillet
Place all but 4 slices of lemon in the skillet.
Sprinkle the bok choy with the black pepper.
Stir fry the bok-choy with the lemons.
Remove and place on four plates.
Place the butter in the skillet and stir fry the salmon, turning once.
Place the salmon on the bed of bok-choy.
Divide the red peppers and encircle the salmon.
Place a slice of lemon atop the salmon.
Drizzle with sriracha sauce.

Nutrition :
Calories 405
Fat: 27g
Protein: 28g
Carbs: 6g

320.   Sriracha Tuna Kabobs

Prep Time : 5 mins
Cook Time : 9 mins
Servings : 4
Ingredients :

4 T Huy Fong chili garlic sauce
1 T sesame oil infused with garlic
1 T ginger, fresh, grated
1 T garlic, minced
1 red onion, cut into quarters and separated by petals
2 cups bell peppers, red, green, yellow
1 can whole water chestnuts, cut in half
½ pound fresh mushrooms, halved
32 oz. boneless tuna, chunks or steaks
1 Splenda packet
2 zucchini, sliced 1 inch thick, keep skins on

Directions :

Layer the tuna and the vegetable pieces evenly onto 8 skewers.
Combine the spices and the oil and chili sauce, add the Splenda
Quickly blend, either in blender or by quickly whipping.
Brush onto the kabob pieces, make sure every piece is coated
Grill 4 minutes on each side, check to ensure the tuna is cooked to taste.
Serving size is two skewers.

Nutrition : Calories 465; Fat: 16g ;Protein: 54g; Carbs: 20g

321.   Brown Basmati Rice Pilaf

Prep Time : 12 mins
Cook Time : 3 mins
Servings : 2
Ingredients :

½ tablespoon vegan butter
½ cup mushrooms, chopped
½ cup brown basmati rice
2-3 tablespoons water
1/8 teaspoon dried thyme
Ground pepper to taste
½ tablespoon olive oil
¼ cup green onion, chopped
1 cup vegetable broth
¼ teaspoon salt
¼ cup chopped, toasted pecans

Directions :

Place a saucepan over medium-low heat. Add butter and oil.

When it melts, add mushrooms and cook until slightly tender.

Stir in the green onion and brown rice. Cook for 3 minutes. Stir constantly.

Stir in the broth, water, salt, and thyme. When it begins to boil, lower the heat and cover with a lid. Simmer until rice is cooked. Add more water or broth if required.

Stir in the pecans and pepper. Serve.

Nutrition :

Calories 185

Fat 10 g

Proteins 4 g

322.   Steak Salad with Asian Spice

Prep Time : 5 mins

Cook Time : 4 mins

Servings : 2

Ingredients :

2 T sriracha sauce

1 T garlic, minced

1 T ginger, fresh, grated

1 bell pepper, yellow, cut in thin strips

1 bell pepper, red, cut in thin strips

1 T sesame oil, garlic

1 Splenda packet

½ teaspoon curry powder

½ teaspoon rice wine vinegar

oz. of beef sirloin, cut into strips

2 cups baby spinach, stemmed

½ head butter lettuce, torn or chopped into bite-sized pieces

Directions :

Place the garlic, sriracha sauce, 1 teaspoon sesame oil, rice wine vinegar, and Splenda into a bowl and combine well.

Pour half of this mix into a zip-lock bag. Add the steak to marinade while you are preparing the salad.

Assemble the brightly colored salad by layering in two bowls.

Place the baby spinach into the bottom of the bowl. Place the butter lettuce next.

Mix the two peppers and place on top.

Remove the steak from the marinade and discard the liquid and bag.

Heat the sesame oil and quickly stir fry the steak until desired doneness, it should take about 3 minutes.

Place the steak on top of the salad.

Drizzle with the remaining dressing (other half of marinade mix).

Sprinkle sriracha sauce across the salad.

Nutrition:

Calories 347

Fat: 22g

Protein: 27g

Carbs: 6g

323.   Simple Beef Roast

Preparation Time: 12 mins

Cooking Time: 8hours **Servings:** 8

Ingredients:

5 pounds' beef roast

2 tablespoons Italian seasoning

1 cup beef stock

1 tablespoon sweet paprika

3 tablespoons olive oil

Directions:

In your slow cooker, mix all the ingredients, cover and cook on low for 8 hours.

Carve the roast, divide it between plates and serve.

Nutrition: Calories: 385 ; Fat: 24 ; Carbs 0.8; Protein 16.2

324.   Vietnamese Turmeric Fish with Mango and Herbs Sauce

Prep Time : 16 mins

Cook Time : 30 mins

Servings : 4

Ingredients :

For the Fish:

Coconut oil to fry the fish, 2 tablespoons

Fresh codfish, skinless and boneless, 1 ¼ lbs. (cut into 2-inch piece wide)

Pinch of sea salt, to taste

Fish Marinade:

Chinese cooking wine, 1 tablespoon

Turmeric powder, 1 tablespoon

Sea salt, 1 teaspoon

Olive oil, 2 tablespoons

Minced ginger, 2 teaspoons

Mango Dipping Sauce:

Juice of ½ lime

Medium-sized ripe mango, 1

Rice vinegar, 2 tablespoons

Dry red chili pepper, 1 teaspoon (stir in before serving)

Garlic clove, 1

Infused scallion and dill oil

Fresh dill, 2 cups

Scallions, 2 cups (slice into long thin shape)

A pinch of sea salt, to taste.

Toppings:

Nuts (pine or cashew nuts)

Lime juice (as much as you like)

Fresh cilantro (as much as you like)

Directions :

Add all the ingredients under "Mango Dipping Sauce" into your food processor. Blend until you get your preferred consistency.

Add two tablespoons of coconut oil in a large non-stick frying pan and heat over high heat. Once hot, add the pre-marinated fish. Add the slices of the fish into the pan individually. Divide into batches for easy frying, if necessary.

Once you hear a loud sizzle, reduce the heat to medium-high.

Do not move or turn the fish until it turns golden brown on one side; then turn it to the other side to fry, about 5 minutes on each side. Add more coconut oil to the pan if needed. Season with the sea salt.

Transfer the fish to a large plate. You will have some oil left in the frypan, which you will use to make your scallion and dill infused oil.

Using the remaining oil in the frypan, set to medium-high heat, add 2 cups of dill, and 2 cups of scallions. Put off the heat after you have added the dill and scallions. Toss them gently for about 15 seconds, until the dill and scallions have wilted. Add a dash of sea salt to season.

Pour the dill, scallion, and infused oil over the fish. Serve with mango dipping sauce, nuts, lime, and fresh cilantro.

Nutrition:

Calories: 230 Fat: 21 g Protein: 74 g Sugar: 4 g

325.   Air Fryer Asparagus

Prep Time : 6 mins

Cook Time : 8 mins

Servings : 1

Ingredients :

Nutritional yeast

Olive oil non-stick spray

One bunch of asparagus

Directions :

Wash the asparagus. Do not forget to trim off thick, woody ends.

Spray with olive oil spray and sprinkle with yeast.

In your Instant Crisp Air Fryer, lay the asparagus in a singular layer. Set the temperature to 360°F. Limit the time to eight minutes.

Nutrition :

Calories: 15

Fat: 4 g

Protein: 9 g

326.   Avocado Fries

Prep Time : 12 mins

Cook Time : 7 mins

Servings : 1

Ingredients :

One avocado

1/8 tsp. salt

1/4 cup of panko breadcrumbs

Bean liquid (aquafaba) from a 15-ounce can of white or garbanzo beans

Directions :

Peel, pit, and slice up avocado.

Toss salt and breadcrumbs together in a bowl. Place the aquafaba into another bowl.

Dredge slices of avocado first in the aquafaba and then in panko, making sure you are evenly coating.

Place coated avocado slices into a single layer in the Instant Crisp Air Fryer. Set temperature to 390°F and set time to 5 minutes.

Serve with your favorite Keto dipping sauce!

Nutrition :

Calories: 100 Fat: 21g

Protein: 9g

Sugar: 1g

327.   Chicken and Kale Curr y .

Prep Time : 22 mins

Cook Time : 1 hour

Servings : 3

Ingredients :

Boiling water, 250 ml

Skinless and boneless chicken thighs, 7 oz.

Ground turmeric, 2 tablespoons

Olive oil, 1 tablespoon

Red onions, 1 (diced)

Bird's eye chili, 1 (finely chopped)

Freshly chopped ginger, ½ tablespoon

Curry powder, ½ tablespoon

Garlic, 1 ½ cloves (crushed)

Cardamom pods, 1

Tinned coconut milk, light, 100 ml

Chicken stock, 2 cups

Tinned chopped tomatoes, 1 cup

Directions :

Place the chicken thighs in a non-metallic bowl, add one tablespoon of turmeric and one teaspoon of olive oil. Mix together and keep aside to marinate for approx. 30 minutes.

Fry the chicken thighs over medium heat for about 5 minutes until well cooked and brown on all sides. Remove from the pan and set aside.

Add the remaining oil into a frypan on medium heat. Then add the onion, ginger, garlic, and chili. Fry for about 10 minutes until soft.

Add one tablespoon of the turmeric and half a tablespoon of curry powder to the pan and cook for another 2 minutes.

Then add the cardamom pods, coconut milk, tomatoes, and chicken stock. Allow simmering for thirty minutes.

Add the chicken once the sauce has reduced a little into the pan, followed by the kale. Cook until the kale is tender and the chicken is warm enough.

Serve with buckwheat.

Garnish with the chopped coriander.

Nutrition:
Calories: 310 g
Protein: 12 g
Fat: 5 g
Carbohydrate: 21 g

328. Mediterranean Baked Penne

Prep Time : 26 mins
Cook Time : 1hour 20 mins
Servings : 8
Ingredients :
Extra-virgin olive oil, 1 tablespoon
Fine dry breadcrumbs, ½ cup
Small zucchini, 2 (chopped)
Medium eggplant, 1 (chopped)
Medium onion, 1 (chopped)
Red bell pepper, 1 (seeded and chopped)
Celery, 1 stalk (sliced)
Garlic, 1 clove (minced)
Salt and freshly ground pepper to taste
Dry white wine, ¼ cup
Plum tomatoes, 28-ounces (drained and coarsely chopped, juice reserved)
Freshly grated Parmesan cheese, 2 tablespoons
Large eggs, 2 (lightly beaten)
Coarsely grated part-skim mozzarella cheese, 1 ½ cups
Dried penne rig ate or rigatoni, 1 pound

Directions :
Preheat your oven to 375 degrees F. Apply nonstick spray on a 3-quart baking dish. Then coat the dish with ¼ cup of breadcrumbs, tapping out the excess. Heat the oil in a large non-stick skillet over medium-high heat. Then add the onion, celery, bell pepper, eggplant, and zucchini.

Cook for about 10 minutes, occasionally stirring, until smooth. Then add the garlic and cook for another minute. Add the wine, stir and cook for about 2 minutes, long enough for the wine to almost evaporate.

Then add the juice and tomatoes. Bring to a simmer, then cook for about 10 to 15 minutes, until thickened, season with pepper and salt.

Transfer to a large bowl and allow to cool.

Pour water into a pot, add some salt, and then allow to boil. Add the penne into the boiling salted water to cook for about 10 minutes, until al dente.

Drain and rinse the pasta under running water. Toss the pasta with the vegetable mixture, then stir in the mozzarella.

Scoop the pasta mixture and place into the prepared baking dish. Drizzle the broken eggs evenly over the top.

Mix the Parmesan and ¼ cups of breadcrumbs in a small bowl, then sprinkle evenly over the top of the dish.

Place the dish into the oven to bake for about 40 to 50 minutes, until bubbly and golden.

Allow to rest for 10 min before you serve.

Nutrition:
Calories: 370
Protein: 43 g
Fat: 7 g
Sugar: 1 g

329. Bell-Pepper Corn Wrapped in Tortilla

Prep Time : 6 mins
Cook Time : 15 mins
Servings : 1
Ingredients :
1/4 small red bell pepper, chopped
1/4 small yellow onion, diced
1/4 tablespoon water
1/2 cobs grilled corn kernels
One large tortilla
One-piece commercial vegan nuggets, chopped
Mixed greens for garnish

Directions :

Preheat the Instant Crisp Air Fryer to 400°F.

In a skillet heated over medium heat, sauté the vegan nuggets and the onions, bell peppers, and corn kernels. Set aside.

Place filling inside the corn tortillas.

Lock the air fryer lid. Fold the tortillas and place inside the Instant Crisp Air Fryer, cook for 15 minutes until the tortilla wraps are crispy.

Serve with mixed greens on top

Nutrition :

Calories: 545

Fat: 20.5g

Protein: 45g

330.   Prawn Arrabbiata

Prep Time : 36 mins

Cook Time : 30 mins

Servings : 1

Ingredients :

Raw or cooked prawns, 1 cup

Extra virgin olive oil, 1 tablespoon

Buckwheat pasta, ½ cup

Chopped parsley, 1 tablespoon

Celery, ¼ cup (finely chopped)

Tinned chopped tomatoes, 2 cups

Red onion, 1/3 cup (finely chopped)

Garlic clove, 1 (finely chopped)

Extra virgin olive oil, 1 teaspoon

Dried mixed herbs, 1 teaspoon

Bird's eye chili, 1 (finely chopped)

White wine, 2 tablespoons (optional)

Directions :

Add the olive oil into your fry-pan and fry the dried herbs, celery, and onions over medium-low heat for about two minutes.

Increase heat to medium, add the wine and cook for another min.

Add the tomatoes to the pan and allow to simmer for about 30 minutes, over medium-low heat, until you get a nice creamy consistency.

Add a little water if the sauce gets too thick.

While the sauce is cooking, cook the pasta following the instruction on the packet. Drain the water once the pasta is done cooking, toss with the olive oil, and set aside until needed.

If using raw prawns, add them to your sauce and cook for another four minutes, until the prawns turn opaque and pink, then add the parsley. If using

cooked prawns, add them at the same time with the parsley and allow the sauce to boil.

Add the already cooked pasta to the sauce, mix them, and serve.

Nutrition :

Calories: 320

Protein: 17 g

Fat: 2 g

Carbohydrate: 21g

331.   Cauliflower Rice

Prep Time : 6 mins

Cook Time : 20 mins

Servings : 1

Ingredients :

Round 1:

1/2 tsp. turmeric

1/2 cup of diced carrot

1/8 cup of diced onion 1/2 tbsp. low-sodium soy sauce

1/8 block of extra firm tofu

Round 2:

1/2 cup of frozen peas

1/4 minced garlic cloves

1/2 cup of chopped broccoli

1/2 tbsp. minced ginger

1/4 tbsp. rice vinegar

1/4 tsp. toasted sesame oil

1/2 tbsp. reduced-sodium soy sauce

1/2 cup of riced cauliflower

Directions :

Crush tofu in a large bowl and toss with all the Round one ingredient.

Lock the air fryer lid — preheat the Instant Crisp Air Fryer to 370 degrees. Also, set the temperature to 370°F, set time to 10 minutes, and cook 10 minutes, making sure to shake once.

In another bowl, toss ingredients from Round 2 together.

Add Round 2 mixture to Instant Crisp Air Fryer and cook another 10 minutes to shake 5 minutes. Enjoy!

Nutrition : Calories: 65; Fat: 8 g ; Protein: 3 g

332.   Stuffed Bacon Mushrooms

Prep Time : 8 mins

Cook Time : 8 mins

Servings : 1

Ingredients :

1/2 rashers bacon, diced

1/2 onion, diced

119

1/2 bell pepper, diced
1/2 small carrot, diced
2 medium size mushrooms (separate the caps and stalks)
1/4 cup shredded cheddar plus extra for to top
1/4 cup sour cream

Directions :
Chop the mushrooms stalks finely and fry them up with the bacon, onion, pepper, and carrot at 350 ° for 8 minutes.
Also, check when the veggies are tender, stir in the sour cream and the cheese. Keep on the heat until the cheese has melted, and everything is mixed nicely. Now grab the mushroom caps and heap a plop of filling on each one.
Place in the fryer basket and top with a little extra cheese.
Nutrition :
Calories: 282
Fat: 20.3 g
Protein: 8.3 g

333.   Zucchini Omelet

Prep Time : 12 mins
Cook Time : 10 mins
Servings : 1
Ingredients :
1/2 teaspoon butter
1/2 zucchini, julienned
One egg
1/8 teaspoon fresh basil, chopped
1/8 teaspoon red pepper flakes, crushed
Salted and newly ground black pepper, to taste
Directions :
Preheat the Instant Crisp Air Fryer to 355 degrees F.
Melt butter on a medium heat using a skillet.
Add zucchini and cook for about 3-4 minutes.
In a bowl, add the eggs, basil, red pepper flakes, salt, and black pepper and beat well.
Add cooked zucchini and gently stir to combine.
Transfer the mixture into the Instant Crisp Air Fryer pan. Lock the air fryer lid.
Cook for about 10 minutes. Also, you may opt to wait until it is done thoroughly.
Nutrition :
Calories: 280
Fat: 20.3
Protein: 8.5

334.   Cheesy Cauliflower Fritters

Prep Time : 12 mins
Cook Time : 7 mins
Servings : 1
Ingredients :
1/2 cup of chopped parsley
1 cup of Italian breadcrumbs
1/3 cup of shredded mozzarella cheese
1/3 cup of shredded sharp cheddar cheese
One egg
Two minced garlic cloves Three chopped scallions
One head of cauliflower
Directions:
Cut the cauliflower up into florets. Wash well and pat dry. Place into a food processor and pulse 20-30 seconds till it looks like rice.
Place the cauliflower rice in a bowl and mix with pepper, salt, egg, cheeses, breadcrumbs, garlic, and scallions.
With hands, form 15 patties of the mixture, and then add more breadcrumbs if needed.
With olive oil, spritz patties, and put the fitters into your Instant Crisp Air Fryer. Pile it in a single layer. Lock the air fryer lid. Set temperature to 390°F, and set time to 7 minutes, flipping after 7 minutes.
Nutrition :
Calories: 208
Fat: 15
Protein: 6

335.   Zucchini Parmesan Chips

Prep Time : 12 mins
Cook Time : 8 mins
Servings : 1
Ingredients :
1/2 tsp. paprika
1/2 cup of grated parmesan cheese
1/2 cup of Italian breadcrumbs
One lightly beaten egg
Two thinly sliced zucchinis
Directions :
Use a very sharp knife or mandolin slicer to slice the zucchini as thinly as you can. Pat off extra moisture.
Beat the egg with a pinch of pepper and salt and a bit of water.
Combine paprika, cheese, and breadcrumbs in a bowl.
Dip slices of zucchini into the egg mixture and then into breadcrumb mixture. Press gently to coat.

With olive oil cooking spray, mist encrusted zucchini slices. Put into your Instant Crisp Air Fryer in a single layer. Latch the air fryer lid. Set temperature to 350°F and set time to 8 minutes.

Sprinkle with salt and serve with salsa.

Nutrition :

Calories: 210

Fat: 15g

Protein: 15g

Sugar: 0

336.   Crispy Roasted Broccoli

Prep Time : 12 mins

Cook Time : 8 mins

Servings : 1

Ingredients :

1/4 tsp. Masala

1/2 tsp. red chili powder

1/2 tsp. salt

1/4 tsp. turmeric powder

1 tbsp. chickpea flour

1 tbsp. yogurt

1/2-pound broccoli

Directions :

Cut broccoli up into florets. Immerse in a bowl of water with two teaspoons of salt for at least half an hour to remove impurities.

Take out broccoli florets from water and let drain. Wipe down thoroughly.

Mix all other ingredients to create a marinade.

Toss broccoli florets in the marinade. Cover and chill 15-30 minutes.

Preheat the Instant Crisp Air Fryer to 390 degrees. Place marinated broccoli florets into the fryer, lock the air fryer lid, set the temperature to 350°F, and set time to 10 minutes. Florets will be crispy when done.

Nutrition :

Calories: 93

Fat: 1.2 g

Protein: 7 g

Sugar: 4.2 g

337.   Crispy Jalapeno Coins

Prep Time : 12 mins

Cook Time : 5 mins

Servings : 1

Ingredients :

One egg

2/3 tbsp. coconut flour

One sliced and seeded jalapeno

Pinch of garlic powder

Pinch of onion powder

Bit of Cajun seasoning (optional)

Pinch of pepper and salt

Directions :

Ensure your Instant Crisp Air Fryer is preheated to 400 degrees.

Mix all dry ingredients.

Pat jalapeno slices dry. Dip them into the egg wash and then into the dry mixture. Toss to coat thoroughly.

Add coated jalapeno slices to Instant Crisp Air Fryer in a singular layer. Spray with olive oil.

Lock the air fryer lid. Set temperature to 350°F and set time to 5 minutes. Cook just till crispy.

Nutrition :

Calories: 125

Fat: 7g

Protein: 6g

Sugar: 0

338.   Jalapeno Cheese Balls

Prep Time : 12 min

Cook Time : 8 mins

Servings : 1

Ingredients :

1-ounce cream cheese

1/6 cup shredded mozzarella cheese

1/6 cup shredded Cheddar cheese

1/2 jalapeños, finely chopped

1/2 cup breadcrumbs

Two eggs

1/2 cup all-purpose flour

Salt

Pepper

Cooking oil

Directions :

Combine the cream cheese, mozzarella, Cheddar, and jalapeños in a medium bowl. Mix well.

Form the cheese mixture into balls about an inch thick. You may also use a small ice cream scoop. It works well.

Arrange the cheese balls on a sheet pan and place in the freezer for 15 minutes. It will help the cheese balls maintain their shape while frying.

Spray the Instant Crisp Air Fryer basket with cooking oil.

Place the breadcrumbs in a small bowl. In another small bowl, beat the eggs. In the third small bowl, combine the flour with salt and pepper to taste, and mix well.

Remove the cheese balls from the freezer. Plunge the cheese balls in the flour, then the eggs, and then the breadcrumbs.

Place the cheese balls in the Instant Crisp Air Fryer. Spray with cooking oil. Lock the air fryer lid. Cook for 8 minutes.

Open the Instant Crisp Air Fryer and flip the cheese balls. I recommend flipping them instead of shaking, so the balls maintain their form. Cook an additional 4 minutes.

Cool before serving .

Nutrition :

Calories: 95

Fat: 11g

Protein: 26g

Sugar: 0

339.   Beauty   School   Ginger Cucumbers

Prep Time : 12 mins

Cook Time : 5 mins

Servings : 14 slices

Ingredients :

1 sliced cucumber

3 teaspoon rice wine vinegar

1 1/2 tablespoon sugar

1 teaspoon minced ginger

Directions :

Bring all of the above **Ingredients:** together in a mixing bowl, and toss the **Ingredients:** well. Enjoy!

Nutrition : Calories: 207; Fat: 6g; Carbs: 12g; Protein18

340.   Mushroom Salad

Prep Time : 12 mins

Cook Time : 20 mins

Servings : 2

Ingredients :

1 tablespoon butter

1/2-pound cremini mushrooms, chopped

2 tablespoon extra-virgin olive oil

Salt and black pepper to taste

2 bunches arugula

4 slices prosciutto

1 tablespoon apple cider vinegar

4 sundried tomatoes in oil, drained and chopped

Parmesan cheese, shaved

Fresh parsley leaves, chopped

Directions :

Heat a pan with butter and half of the oil.

Add the mushrooms, salt, and pepper. Stir-fry for 3 minutes. Reduce heat. Stir again, and cook for 3 minutes more.

Add rest of the oil and vinegar. Stir and cook for 1 minute.

Place arugula on a platter, add prosciutto on top, add the mushroom mixture, sundried tomatoes, more salt and pepper, parmesan shavings, parsley, and serve.

Nutrition :

Calories: 190

Fat: 6g

Carbs: 5g

Protein 15g

341.   Coconut   Battered Cauliflower Bites

Prep Time : 6 mins

Cook Time : 20 mins

Servings : 1

Ingredients :

Salt and pepper to taste

One flax egg or one tablespoon flaxseed meal + 3 tablespoon water

One small cauliflower, cut into florets

One teaspoon mixed spice

1/2 teaspoon mustard powder

Two tablespoons maple syrup

One clove of garlic, minced

Two tablespoons soy sauce

1/3 cup oats flour

1/3 cup plain flour

1/3 cup desiccated coconut

Directions :

In a mixing bowl, mix oats, flour, and desiccated coconut. Season with salt and pepper to taste. Set aside.

In another bowl, place the flax egg and add a pinch of salt to taste. Set aside.

Season the cauliflower with mixed spice and mustard powder.

Dredge the florets in the flax egg first, then in the flour mixture.

Place it inside the Instant Crisp Air Fryer, lock the air fryer lid, and cook at 400°F or 15 minutes.

Meanwhile, place the maple syrup, garlic, and soy sauce in a saucepan and heat over medium flame.

Wait for it to boil and adjust the heat to low until the sauce thickens.

After 15 minutes, take out the Instant Crisp Air Fryer's florets and place them in the saucepan.

Toss to coat the florets and place inside the Instant Crisp Air Fryer and cook for another 5 minutes.

Nutrition:

Calories: 152

Fat: 2.2

Protein: 4.6

342.   Easy Pork Ribs

Prep Time : 12 mins

Cook Time : 15 mins

Servings : 6

Ingredients :

3 pounds boneless pork ribs

½ cup soy sauce

¼ cup ketchup

2 tablespoons olive oil

Black pepper to taste

Directions :

Pour oil into your PPCXL and hit "chicken/meat," leaving the lid off.

When oil is hot, add ribs and sear till golden on both sides.

In a bowl, mix black pepper, soy sauce, and ketchup.

Pour over ribs and seal the lid.

Adjust cook time to 15 minutes.

When the timer beeps, hit "cancel" and wait 5 minutes before quick-releasing.

Make sure pork is at least 145-degrees before serving.

Nutrition :

Calories: 565

Total Fat: 25g

Total carbs: 0

Fiber: 0

Protein: 62g

343.   Pineapple-BBQ Pork

Prep Time : 12 mins

Cook Time : 6 mins

Servings : 4

Ingredients :

4 bone-in pork loin chops

One 8-ounce can of undrained crushed pineapple

1 cup honey BBQ sauce

2 tablespoons chili sauce

1 tablespoon olive oil

Directions :

Mix can of pineapple, BBQ sauce, and chili sauce.

Turn your PPCXL to "chicken/meat" and heat.

When hot, add olive oil.

When the oil is sizzling, sear pork chops on both sides, 3-4 minutes per side.

When brown, pour sauce over the pork and seal the lid.

Adjust time to 6 minutes.

When time is up, hit "cancel" and wait 5 minutes before quick-releasing.

Pork should be cooked to 145-degrees.

Serve with sauce.

Nutrition :

Calories: 367

Protein: 25

Total Fat: 12

Carbs: 35

Fiber: 0

344.   Apple-Garlic Pork Loin

Prep Time : 6 mins

Cook Time : 25 mins

Servings : 12

Ingredients :

One 3-pound boneless pork loin roast

One 12-ounce jar of apple jelly

1/3 cup water

1 tablespoon Herbs de Provence

2 teaspoons minced garlic

Directions :

Put pork loin in your cooker. Cut in half if necessary.

Mix garlic, water, and jelly.

Pour over pork.

Season with Herbs de Provence.

Seal the lid.

Hit "chicken/meat" and adjust time to 25 minutes.

When time is up, hit "cancel" and wait 10 minutes before quick-releasing.

Pork should be served at 145-degrees. If not cooked through yet, hit "chicken/meat" and cook with the lid off until temperature is reached.

Rest for 15 minutes before slicing.

Nutrition :

Calories: 232

Total Fat: 6

Total carbs: 16

Protein: 25

345. Pork with Cranberry - Honey Gravy

Prep Time : 12 mins
Cook Time : 72 mins
Servings : 4
Ingredients :
2 ½ pounds bone-in pork shoulder
One 15-ounce can of whole-berry cranberry sauce
¼ cup minced onion
¼ cup honey
Salt to taste
Directions :
Add all the ingredients into your pressure cooker and seal the lid.
Hit "chicken/meat" and adjust time to 1 hour, 12 minutes.
When time is up, hit "cancel" and wait 10 minutes for a natural pressure release.
Remove the shoulder and de-bone.
Serve pork with gravy!
Nutrition :
Calories: 704 Total Fat: 27
Total carbs: 60
Protein: 41
Fiber: 0

346. Mexican-Braised Pork with Sweet Potatoes

Prep Time : 12 mins
Cook Time : 25 mins
Servings : 4
Ingredients :
3 pounds pork loin
2 peeled and diced sweet potatoes
1 cup tomato salsa
½ cup chicken stock
1/3 cup Mexican spice blend
Directions :
Season the pork all over with the spice blend.
Turn your cooker to "chicken/meat" and heat.
When hot, sear the pork on both sides. If the meat sticks, pour in a little chicken stock.
When the pork is golden, pour in stock and salsa.
Tumble sweet potatoes on one side of the pot and seal the lid.
Adjust time to 25 minutes.
When the timer beeps, hit "cancel" and wait 10 minutes before quick-releasing.
The pork should be cooked to 145-degrees, and the potatoes should be tender.

Remove the pork and rest 8-10 minutes before serving.
Nutrition:
Calories: 510
Total Fat: 13
Protein: 71
carbs: 16

347. Peach-Mustard Pork Shoulder

Prep Time : 3 min
Cook Time : 55 Mins
Servings : 8
Ingredients:
4 pounds pork shoulder
1 cup peach preserving:
1 cup white wine
1/3 cup salt
1 tablespoon grainy mustard
Directions :
Season the pork well with salt.
Mix mustard and peach, and rub on the pork.
Pour wine into cooker and add pork.
Seal the lid.
Hit "chicken/meat" and adjust time to 55 minutes.
When time is up, hit "cancel" and wait 10 minutes before quick-releasing.
Pork should be cooked to at least 145-degrees.
Move pork to a plate and tent with foil for 15 minutes before slicing and serving.
Nutrition:
Calories: 580 Fat: 30
Carbs: 25 Protein: 43

348. Balsamic Beef and Mushrooms Mix

Preparation Time : 6 mins
Cook Time : 8 mins
Servings: 4
Ingredients:
2 pounds' beef, cut into strips
¼ cup balsamic vinegar
2 cups beef stock
1 tablespoon ginger, grated
Juice of ½ lemon
1 cup brown mushrooms, sliced
A pinch of salt and black pepper
1 teaspoon ground cinnamon
Directions:

Mix all the ingredients in your slow cooker, cover and cook on low for 8 hours.

Divide everything between plates and serve.

Nutrition:

Calories: 445

Fat: 13

Fiber 0.5

Carbs 2.8

Protein 70.6

349. Oregano Pork Mix

Preparation Time : 6 mins

Cook Time : 7h 6 minutes

Servings: 4

Ingredients:

2 pounds' pork roast

7 ounces' tomato paste

1 yellow onion, chopped

1 cup beef stock

2 tablespoons ground cumin

2 tablespoons olive oil

2 tablespoons fresh oregano, chopped

1 tablespoon garlic, minced

½ cup fresh thyme, chopped

Directions:

Heat up a sauté pan with the oil over medium-high heat, add the roast, brown it for 3 minutes on each side and then transfer to your slow cooker.

Add the rest of the ingredients, toss a bit, cover and cook on low for 7 hours.

Slice the roast, divide it between plates and serve.

Nutrition :

Calories: 620 Fat: 30

Fiber 6 Carbs 19

Protein 69

350. Chicken Breast Soup

Preparation Time: 6 min

Cooking Time: 4 hours

Servings: 4

Ingredients:

3 chicken breasts, skinless, boneless, cubed

2 celery stalks, chopped

2 carrots, chopped

2 tablespoons olive oil

1 red onion, chopped

3 garlic cloves, minced

4 cups chicken stock

1 tablespoon parsley, chopped

Directions:

In your slow cooker, mix all the ingredients except the parsley, cover and cook on High for 4 hours.

Add the parsley, stir, ladle the soup into bowls and serve.

Nutrition:

Calories: 440

Fat: 21

Fiber 1.3

Carbs 7.2

Protein 54

351. Cauliflower Curry

Preparation Time: 6 minutes

Cook Time: 5 hours

Servings: 4

Ingredients:

1 cauliflower head, florets separated

2 carrots, sliced

1 red onion, chopped

¾ cup coconut milk

2 garlic cloves, minced

2 tablespoons curry powder

A pinch of salt and black pepper

1 tablespoon red pepper flakes

1 teaspoon garam masala

Directions:

In your slow cooker, mix all the ingredients.

Cover, cook on high for 5 hours, divide into bowls and serve.

Nutrition:

Calories: 155

Fat: 11.2

Fiber 5.3

Carbs 14.4

Protein 3.2

352. Pork and Peppers Chili

Preparation Time: 6 minutes

Cooking Time: 8 hours 5 min

Servings: 4

Ingredients:

1 red onion, chopped

2 pounds' pork, ground

4 garlic cloves, minced

2 red bell peppers, chopped

1 celery stalk, chopped

25 ounces' fresh tomatoes, peeled, crushed

¼ cup green chilies, chopped

2 tablespoons fresh oregano, chopped

125

2 tablespoons chili powder

A pinch of salt and black pepper

A drizzle of olive oil

Directions:

Heat up a sauté pan with the oil over medium-high heat and add the onion, garlic and the meat. Mix and brown for 5 minutes then transfer to your slow cooker.

Add the rest of the ingredients, toss, cover and cook on low for 8 hours.

Divide everything into bowls and serve.

Nutrition:

Calories: 440

Fat: 12

Fiber 6.4

Carbs 20

Protein 62

353.   Greek Style Quesadillas

Preparation Time: 12 minutes

Cooking Time : 10 minutes **Servings:** 4

Ingredients:

4 whole wheat tortillas

1 cup Mozzarella cheese, shredded

1 cup fresh spinach, chopped

2 tablespoon Greek yogurt

1 egg, beaten

¼ cup green olives, sliced

1 tablespoon olive oil

1/3 cup fresh cilantro, chopped

Directions:

In the bowl, combine together Mozzarella cheese, spinach, yogurt, egg, olives, and cilantro.

Then pour olive oil in the skillet.

Place one tortilla in the skillet and spread it with Mozzarella mixture.

Top it with the second tortilla and spread it with cheese mixture again.

Then place the third tortilla and spread it with all remaining cheese mixture.

Cover it with the last tortilla and fry it for 5 minutes from each side over the medium heat.

Nutrition:

Calories: 191

Fat: 7.2

Fiber 3

Carbs 23.4

Protein 8.2

354.   Creamy Penne

Preparation Time : 12 min

Cooking Time : 25 min

Servings : 4

Ingredients:

½ cup penne, dried

oz. chicken fillet

1 teaspoon Italian seasoning

1 tablespoon olive oil

1 tomato, chopped

1 cup heavy cream

1 tablespoon fresh basil, chopped

½ teaspoon salt

2 oz. Parmesan, grated

1 cup water, for cooking

Directions:

Pour water in the pan, add penne, and boil it for 15 minutes. Then drain water.

Pour olive oil in the skillet and heat it up.

Slice the chicken fillet and put it in the hot oil.

Sprinkle chicken with Italian seasoning and roast for 2 minutes from each side.

Then add fresh basil, salt, tomato, and grated cheese. Stir well.

Add heavy cream and cooked penne.

Cook the meal for 5 minutes

Nutrition:

Calories: 385

Fat: 23.2

Fiber 0.1

Carbs 17.3

Protein 17.5

355.   Light Paprika Moussaka

Preparation Time: 16 min

Cooking Time : 45 min

Servings: 3

Ingredients:

1 eggplant, trimmed

1 cup ground chicken

1/3 cup white onion, diced

3 oz. Cheddar cheese, shredded

1 potato, sliced

1 teaspoon olive oil

1 teaspoon salt

½ cup milk

1 tablespoon butter

1 tablespoon ground paprika

1 tablespoon Italian seasoning

1 teaspoon tomato paste

Directions:
Slice the eggplant lengthwise and sprinkle with salt.
Pour olive oil in the skillet and add sliced potato.
Roast potato for 2 minutes from each side.
Then transfer it in the plate.
Put eggplant in the skillet and roast it for 2 minutes from each side too.
Pour milk in the pan and bring it to boil.
Add tomato paste, Italian seasoning, paprika, butter, and Cheddar cheese.
Then mix up together onion with ground chicken.
Arrange the sliced potato in the casserole in one layer.
Then add ½ part of all sliced eggplants.
Spread the eggplants with ½ part of chicken mixture.
Then add remaining eggplants.
Pour the milk mixture over the eggplants.
Bake moussaka for 30 minutes at 355F.

Nutrition:
Calories: 385
Fat: 21
Fiber 8.5
Carbs 26.2
Protein 25.2

356. Cucumber Bowl with Spices and Greek Yogurt

Preparation Time : 12 min
Cooking Time : 20 min
Servings: 3
Ingredients:
4 cucumbers
½ teaspoon chili pepper
¼ cup fresh parsley, chopped
¾ cup fresh dill, chopped
2 tablespoons lemon juice
½ teaspoon salt
½ teaspoon ground black pepper
¼ teaspoon sage
½ teaspoon dried oregano
1/3 cup Greek yogurt

Directions:
Make the cucumber dressing: blend the dill and parsley until you get green mash.
Then combine together green mash with lemon juice, salt, ground black pepper, sage, dried oregano, Greek yogurt, and chili pepper.
Churn the mixture well.
Chop the cucumbers roughly and combine them with cucumber dressing. Mix up well.
Refrigerate the cucumber for 20 minutes.

Nutrition:
Calories: 110
Fat: 1.5
Fiber 4
Carbs 23
Protein 7.2

357. Stuffed Bell Peppers with Quinoa

Preparation Time : 12 minutes Cooking Time : 35 minutes **Servings :** 2
Ingredients:
2 bell peppers
1/3 cup quinoa
3 oz. chicken stock
¼ cup onion, diced
½ teaspoon salt
¼ teaspoon tomato paste
½ teaspoon dried oregano
1/3 cup sour cream
1 teaspoon paprika

Directions:
Trim the bell peppers and remove the seeds.
Then combine together chicken stock and quinoa in the pan.
Add salt and boil the ingredients for 10 minutes or until quinoa will soak all liquid.
Then combine together cooked quinoa with dried oregano, tomato paste, and onion.
Fill the bell peppers with the quinoa mixture and arrange in the casserole mold.
Add sour cream and bake the peppers for 25 minutes at 365F.
Serve the cooked peppers with sour cream sauce from the casserole mold.

Nutrition:
Calories 232
Fat 10
Carbs 31
Protein 6.6

358. Mediterranean Burrito

Preparation Time : 12 minutes Cooking Time : 0 minutes **Servings:** 2
Ingredients:
2 wheat tortillas
2 oz. red kidney beans, canned, drained
2 tablespoons hummus
2 teaspoons tahini sauce
1 cucumber

2 lettuce leaves

1 tablespoon lime juice

1 teaspoon olive oil

½ teaspoon dried oregano

Directions:

Mash the red kidney beans until you get a puree.

Then spread the wheat tortillas with beans mash from one side.

Add hummus and tahini sauce.

Cut the cucumber into the wedges and place them over tahini sauce.

Then add lettuce leaves.

Make the dressing: mix up together olive oil, dried oregano, and lime juice.

Drizzle the lettuce leaves with the dressing and wrap the wheat tortillas in the shape of burritos.

Nutrition:

Calories 280

Fat 10g

Carbs 38g

Fiber 14g

Protein 12g

359. Sweet Potato Bacon Mash

Preparation Time : 12 minutes Cooking Time : 20 minutes **Servings:** 4

Ingredients:

3 sweet potatoes, peeled

4 oz. bacon, chopped

1 cup chicken stock

1 tablespoon butter

1 teaspoon salt

2 oz. Parmesan, grated

Directions:

Chop sweet potato and put it in the pan.

Add chicken stock and close the lid.

Boil the vegetables for 15 minutes or until they are soft.

After this, drain the chicken stock.

Mash the sweet potato with the help of the potato masher. Add grated cheese and butter.

Mix up together salt and chopped bacon. Fry the mixture until it is crunchy (10-15 minutes).

Add cooked bacon in the mashed sweet potato and mix up with the help of the spoon.

It is recommended to serve the meal warm or hot.

Nutrition:

Calories 300 Fat 18g

Carbs 18.4g

Fiber 2.6g Protein 17g

360. Prosciutto Wrapped Mozzarella Balls

Preparation Time: 12 minutes Cooking Time : 10 minutes **Servings:** 4

Ingredients:

Mozzarella balls, cherry size

4 oz. bacon, sliced

¼ teaspoon ground black pepper

¾ teaspoon dried rosemary

1 teaspoon butter

Directions:

Sprinkle the sliced bacon with ground black pepper and dried rosemary.

Wrap every Mozzarella ball in the sliced bacon and secure them with toothpicks.

Melt butter.

Brush wrapped Mozzarella balls with butter.

Line the tray with the baking paper and arrange Mozzarella balls in it.

Bake the meal for 10 minutes at 365F.

Nutrition:

Calories: 320

Fat: 26.4 g

Fiber: 0.1

Carbs: 0.5 g

Protein: 20.2 g

361. Garlic Chicken Balls

Preparation Time : 16 minutes Cooking Time : 10 minutes **Servings:** 4

Ingredients :

2 cups ground chicken

1 teaspoon minced garlic

1 teaspoon dried dill

1/3 carrot, grated

1 egg, beaten

1 tablespoon olive oil

¼ cup coconut flakes

½ teaspoon salt

Directions:

In the mixing bowl mix up together ground chicken, minced garlic, dried dill, carrot, egg, and salt.

Stir the chicken mixture with the help of the fingertips until homogenous.

Then make medium balls from the mixture.

Coat every chicken ball in coconut flakes.

Heat up olive oil in the skillet.

Add chicken balls and cook them for 3 minutes from each side.

The cooked chicken balls will have a golden-brown color.

Nutrition:
Calories: 195
Fat: 11.3
Fiber 0.5
Carbs 1.5
Protein 21.7

362.   Zucchini Salmon Salad

Preparation Time : 6 min Cooking Time : 10 minutes
Servings : 3
Ingredients :
2 salmon fillets
2 tablespoons soy sauce
2 zucchinis, sliced
Salt and pepper to taste
2 tablespoons extra virgin olive oil
2 tablespoons sesame seeds
Salt and pepper to taste
Directions:
Drizzle the salmon with soy sauce.
Heat a grill pan over medium flame. Cook salmon on the grill on each side for 2-3 minutes.
Season the zucchini with salt and pepper and place it on the grill as well. Cook on each side until golden.
Place the zucchini, salmon and the rest of the ingredients in a bowl.
Serve the salad fresh.
Nutrition:
Calories: 220
Fat: 18 g
Carbs: 0 g
Protein: 18 g

363.   Homemade Vegetable Broth

Preparation Time : 6 minutes Cooking Time : 30 minutes **Servings : 4**
Ingredients :
1 tablespoon olive oil
1 chopped onion
2 chopped stalks celery
2 chopped carrots
1 head bok choy
6 cups or 1 package fresh spinach
2+ quarts of water
1 tablespoon salt
½ teaspoon pepper
1 teaspoon fresh sage

Directions :
Sauté vegetables in oil. Add water and simmer for 1 hour.
Keep adding water as needed.
Pour broth mixture into pint and quart mason jars.
Leave one full inch of space from the top of the jar or it will crack when it freezes as liquids expand.
Place jars in freezer for up to a year.
Take out and use whenever you make a soup.
Nutrition :
Calories: 138
Fat: 2g
Fiber: 22g
Carbs: 21g
Protein: 45g

364.   Mediterranean   Chickpea Salad

Prep Time : 6 Minutes
Cook Time: 20 Minutes **Servings:** 6
Ingredients :
1 can chickpeas, drained
1 fennel bulb, sliced
1 red onion, sliced
1 teaspoon dried basil
1 teaspoon dried oregano
2 tablespoons chopped parsley
4 garlic cloves, minced
2 tablespoons lemon juice
2 tablespoons extra virgin olive oil
Salt and pepper to taste
Directions:
Combine the chickpeas, fennel, red onion, herbs, garlic, lemon juice and oil in a salad bowl.
Add salt and pepper and serve the salad fresh.
Nutrition:
Calories 198
Fat 8g
Carbs 28g
Protein 4g

365.   Warm   Chorizo   Chickpea Salad

Prep Time : 6 Minutes
Cook Time : 20 Minutes
Servings: 6
Ingredients :
1 tablespoon extra-virgin olive oil
4 chorizo links, sliced
1 red onion, sliced

4 roasted red bell peppers, chopped
1 can chickpeas, drained
2 cups cherry tomatoes
2 tablespoons balsamic vinegar
Salt and pepper to taste

Directions:

Heat the oil in a skillet and add the chorizo. Cook briefly just until fragrant then add the onion, bell peppers and chickpeas and cook for 2 additional minutes.

Transfer the mixture in a salad bowl then add the tomatoes, vinegar, salt and pepper.

Mix well and serve the salad right away.

Nutrition :
Calories 350
Fat 17g
Carbs 20g
Protein 14g

366. Greek Roasted Fish

Prep Time: 6 Minutes
Cook Time: 30 Minutes
Servings: 4
Ingredients:
4 salmon fillets
1 tablespoon chopped oregano
1 teaspoon dried basil
1 zucchini, sliced
1 red onion, sliced
1 carrot, sliced
1 lemon, sliced
2 tablespoons extra virgin olive oil
Salt and pepper to taste

Directions :

add all the ingredients in a deep dish baking pan.

Season with salt and pepper and cook in the preheated oven at 350F for 20 minutes.

Serve the fish and vegetables warm.

Nutrition :
Calories 325 Fat 12g
Carbs 8g Protein 36g

367. Garlicky Tomato Chicken Casserole

Prep Time : 6 Minutes
Cook Time : 50 Minutes
Servings : 4
Ingredients :
4 chicken breasts
2 tomatoes, sliced

1 can diced tomatoes
2 garlic cloves, chopped
1 shallot, chopped
1 bay leaf
1 thyme sprig
½ cup dry white wine
½ cup chicken stock
Salt and pepper to taste

Directions :

Combine the chicken and the remaining ingredients in a deep dish baking pan.

Adjust the taste with salt and pepper and cover the pot with a lid or aluminum foil.

Cook in the preheated oven at 330F for 40 minutes.

Serve the casserole warm.

Nutrition :
Calories 310 Fat 7g
Carbs 6g Protein 45g

368. Chicken Cacciatore

Preparation Time : 6 minutes
Cooking Time: 45 minutes
Servings: 6
Ingredients:
2 tablespoons extra virgin olive oil
6 chicken thighs
1 sweet onion, chopped
2 garlic cloves, minced
2 red bell peppers, cored and diced
2 carrots, diced
1 rosemary sprig
1 thyme sprig
4 tomatoes, peeled and diced
½ cup tomato juice
¼ cup dry white wine
1 cup chicken stock
1 bay leaf
Salt and pepper to taste

Directions:

Heat the oil in a heavy saucepan.

Cook chicken on all sides until golden.

Stir in the onion and garlic and cook for 2 minutes.

Stir in the rest of the ingredients and season with salt and pepper.

Cook on low heat for 30 minutes. Serve the chicken cacciatore warm and fresh.

Nutrition:

Calories 360 Fat 13 g
Carbs 9g
Protein 41g

369. Fennel Wild Rice Risotto

Preparation Time : 6 min
Cooking Time: 35minutes
Servings : 6
Ingredients:
2 tablespoons extra virgin olive oil
1 shallot, chopped
2 garlic cloves, minced
1 fennel bulb, chopped
1 cup wild rice
¼ cup dry white wine
2 cups chicken stock
1 teaspoon grated orange zest
Salt and pepper to taste
Directions:
Heat the oil in a heavy saucepan.
Add the garlic, shallot and fennel and cook for a few minutes until softened.
Stir in the rice and cook for 2 additional minutes then add the wine, stock and orange zest, with salt and pepper to taste.
Cook on low heat for 20 minutes.
Serve the risotto warm and fresh.
Nutrition:
Calories 160
Fat 2 g
Carbs 18 g
Protein 7 g

370. Wild Rice Prawn Salad

Preparation Time : 6 minutes
Cooking Time : 35 minutes
Servings : 6
Ingredients:
¾ cup wild rice
1¾ cups chicken stock
1 pound prawns
Salt and pepper to taste
2 tablespoons lemon juice
2 tablespoons extra virgin olive oil
2 cups arugula
Directions:
Combine the rice and chicken stock in a saucepan and cook until the liquid has been absorbed entirely.
Transfer the rice in a salad bowl.
Season the prawns with salt and pepper and drizzle them with lemon juice and oil.
Heat a grill pan over medium flame.
Place the prawns on the hot pan and cook on each side for 2-3 minutes.

For the salad, combine the rice with arugula and prawns and mix well.
Serve the salad fresh.
Nutrition:
Calories 205
Fat 4 g
Protein 20.5 g
Carbs 15g

371. Chicken Broccoli Salad with Avocado Dressing

Preparation Time : 6
Cooking Time: 40 minutes
Servings : 6
Ingredients:
2 chicken breasts
1 pound broccoli, cut into florets
1 avocado, peeled and pitted
½ lemon, juiced
2 garlic cloves
¼ teaspoon chili powder
¼ teaspoon cumin powder
Salt and pepper to taste
Directions:
Cook the chicken in a large pot of salty water.
Drain and cut the chicken into small cubes. Place in a salad bowl.
Add the broccoli and mix well.
Combine the avocado, lemon juice, garlic, chili powder, cumin powder, salt and pepper in a blender. Pulse until smooth.
Spoon the dressing over the salad and mix well.
Serve the salad fresh.
Nutrition :
Calories 190
Fat 10 g
Carbs 3 g
Protein 14 g

372. Seafood Paella

Preparation Time: 6 minutes
Cooking Time : 45 minutes **Servings :** 8
Ingredients:
2 tablespoons extra virgin olive oil
1 shallot, chopped
2 garlic cloves, chopped
1 red bell pepper, cored and diced
1 carrot, diced
2 tomatoes, peeled and diced
1 cup wild rice

1 cup tomato juice

2 cups chicken stock

1 chicken breast, cubed

Salt and pepper to taste

2 monkfish fillets, cubed

½ pound fresh shrimps, peeled and deveined

½ pound prawns

1 thyme sprig

1 rosemary sprig

Directions:

Heat the oil in a skillet and stir in the shallot, garlic, bell pepper, carrot and tomatoes. Cook for a few minutes until softened.

Stir in the rice, tomato juice, stock, chicken, salt and pepper and cook on low heat for 20 minutes.

Add the rest of the ingredients and cook for 10 additional minutes.

Serve the paella warm and fresh.

Nutrition: Calories: 243; Fat: 7g ; Protein: 26g; Carbs: 20.4g

373. Mu Shu Lunch Pork

Preparation Time : 6 minutes Cooking Time : 10 minutes **Servings:** 2

Ingredients:

4 cups coleslaw mix, with carrots

1 small onion, sliced thin

1 lb. cooked roast pork, cut into ½" cubes

2 tbsp. hoisin sauce

2 tbsp. soy sauce

Directions:

In a large skillet, heat the oil on a high heat.

Stir-fry the cabbage and onion for 4 minutes until tender.

Add the pork, hoisin and soy sauce.

Cook until browned.

Nutrition :

Calories: 385

Carbs: 15 g

Fat: 20 g

Protein: 25 g

374. Courgette Risotto

Preparation Time : 12 minutes Cooking Time : 5 minutes **Servings :** 8

Ingredients :

2 tablespoons olive oil

4 cloves garlic, finely chopped

1.5 pounds Arborio rice

6 tomatoes, chopped

2 teaspoons chopped rosemary

6 courgettes, finely diced

1 ¼ cups peas, fresh or frozen

cups hot vegetable stock

Salt to taste

Freshly ground pepper

Directions:

Place a large, heavy-bottomed pan over medium heat. Add oil. When the oil is heated, add onion and sauté until translucent.

Stir in the tomatoes and cook until soft.

Stir in the rice and rosemary. Mix well.

Add half the stock and cook until dry. Stir frequently.

Add remaining stock and cook for 3-4 minutes.

Add courgette and peas and cook until rice is tender.

Add salt and pepper to taste.

Stir in the basil. Let it sit for 5 minutes.

Nutrition:

Calories 403

Fats 5 g

Carbohydrates 80g

375. Proteins 12 g

Instant Pot Chipotle Chicken & Cauliflower Rice Bowls

Preparation Time: 12min

Cooking Time: 20 min **Servings:** 4

Ingredients :

1/3 cup of salsa

1 quantity of 14.5 oz. of can fire-roasted diced tomatoes

1 canned chipotle pepper + 1 teaspoon sauce

½ teaspoon of dried oregano

1 teaspoon of cumin

1 ½ lb. of boneless, skinless chicken breast

¼ teaspoon of salt

1 cup of reduced-fat shredded Mexican cheese blend

4 cups of frozen riced cauliflower

½ medium-sized avocado, sliced

Directions:

Combine the first ingredients in a blender and blend until they become smooth

Place chicken inside your instant pot, and pour the sauce over it. Cover the lid and close the pressure valve.

Set it to 20 minutes at high temperature. Let the pressure release on its own before opening.

Remove the piece and the chicken and then add it back to the sauce.

Microwave the riced cauliflower according to the directions on the package.

Before you serve, divide the riced cauliflower, cheese, avocado, and chicken equally among the four bowls.

Nutrition:
Calories: 285
Protein: 34 g
Carbohydrate: 18 g
Fat: 11 g

376. Homemade Chicken Broth

Preparation Time : 6 minutes Cooking Time : 30 minutes **Servings :** 4
Ingredients :
1 tablespoon olive oil
1 chopped onion
2 chopped stalks celery
2 chopped carrots
1 whole chicken
2+ quarts of water
1 tablespoon salt
½ teaspoon pepper
1 teaspoon fresh sage

Directions :
Sauté vegetables in oil.

Add chicken and water and simmer for 2+ hours until the chicken falls off the bone. Keep adding water as needed.

Remove the chicken carcass from the broth, place on a platter, and let it cool. Pull chicken off the carcass and put it into the broth.

Pour broth mixture into pint and quart mason jars. Be sure to add meat to each jar.

Leave one full inch of space from the top of the jar or it will crack when it freezes as liquids expand. Place jars in freezer for up to a year.

Take out and use whenever you make a soup.

Nutrition :
Calories: 210
Fat: 6g
Carbs: 15g
Protein: 21g

377. Grilled Salmon with Pineapple Salsa

Prep Time: 6 Minutes
Cook Time: 30 Minutes **Servings:** 4
Ingredients
4 salmon fillets
Salt and pepper to taste
2 tablespoons Cajun seasoning
1 fresh pineapple, peeled and diced
1 cup cherry tomatoes, quartered
2 tablespoons chopped cilantro
2 tablespoons chopped parsley
1 teaspoon dried mint
2 tablespoons lemon juice
2 tablespoons extra virgin olive oil
1 teaspoon honey
Salt and pepper to taste

Directions :
Add salt, pepper and Cajun seasoning to the fish.

Heat a grill pan over medium flame. Cook fish on the grill on each side for 3-4 minutes.

For the salsa, mix the pineapple, tomatoes, cilantro, parsley, mint, lemon juice and honey in a bowl. Season with salt and pepper.

Serve the grilled salmon with the pineapple salsa.

Nutrition:
Calories 330
Fat 11g
Carbs 7
Protein 33

378. Fish Stew

Preparation Time : 6 minutes Cooking Time : 30 minutes **Servings:** 4
Ingredients :
1 tablespoon olive oil
1 chopped onion or leek
2 chopped stalks celery
2 chopped carrots
1 clove minced garlic
1 tablespoon parsley
1 bay leaf
1 clove
1/8 teaspoon kelp or dulse (seaweed)
¼ teaspoon salt
Fish—leftover, cooked, diced
2–3 cups chicken or vegetable broth

Directions:
Add all of ingredients and simmer on the stove for 20 minutes.

Nutrition:
Calories: 340
Fat: 14g
Fiber: 10g
Carbs: 8g
Protein: 10g

379.   Pan Fried Salmon

Preparation Time : 6 minutes Cooking Time : 20 minutes **Servings:** 4

Ingredients :

4 salmon fillets

Salt and pepper to taste

1 teaspoon dried oregano

1 teaspoon dried basil

3 tablespoons extra virgin olive oil

Directions:

Season the fish with salt, pepper, oregano and basil. Heat the oil in a pan and place the salmon in the hot oil, with the skin facing down.

Fry on each side for 2 minutes until golden brown and fragrant.

Serve the salmon warm and fresh.

Nutrition:

Calories: 325

Fat: 24g

Protein: 35g

Carbohydrates: 0.3g

380.   Tomato Fish Bake

Preparation Time : 6 minutes Cooking Time : 30 minutes **Servings** : 4

Ingredients :

4 cod fillets

4 tomatoes, sliced

4 garlic cloves, minced

1 shallot, sliced

1 celery stalk, sliced

1 teaspoon fennel seeds

1 cup vegetable stock

Salt and pepper to taste

Directions:

Layer the cod fillets and tomatoes in a deep dish baking pan.

Add the rest of the ingredients and add salt and pepper.

Cook in the preheated oven at 350F for 20 minutes.

Serve the dish warm or chilled.

Nutrition:

Calories: 297

Fat: 3g

Protein: 62g

Carbohydrates: 2g

381.   Herbed Roasted Chicken Breasts

Preparation Time : 6 minutes Cooking Time : 50 minutes **Servings:** 4

Ingredients :

2 tablespoons extra virgin olive oil

2 tablespoons chopped parsley

2 tablespoons chopped cilantro

1 teaspoon dried oregano

1 teaspoon dried basil

2 tablespoons lemon juice

Salt and pepper to taste

4 chicken breasts

Directions:

Combine the oil, parsley, cilantro, oregano, basil, lemon juice, salt and pepper in a bowl.

Spread this mixture over the chicken and rub it well into the meat.

Place in a deep dish baking pan and cover with aluminum foil.

Cook in the preheated oven at 350F for 20 minutes then remove the foil and cook for 25 additional minutes.

Serve the chicken warm and fresh with your favorite side dish.

Nutrition:

Calories: 327

Fat: 14g

Protein: 40g

Carbohydrates: 1g

382.   Marinated Chicken Breasts

Preparation Time : 6 minutes Cooking Time : 2 hours **Servings:** 4

Ingredients :

4 chicken breasts

Salt and pepper to taste

1 lemon, juiced

1 rosemary sprig

1 thyme sprig

2 garlic cloves, crushed

2 sage leaves

3 tablespoons extra virgin olive oil

½ cup buttermilk

Directions :

Boil the chicken with salt and pepper and place it in a resealable bag.

Add remaining ingredients and seal bag.

Refrigerate for at least 1 hour.

After 1 hour, heat a roasting pan over medium heat, then place the chicken on the grill.

Cook on each side for 8-10 minutes or until juices are gone.

Serve the chicken warm with your favorite side dish.

Nutrition:

Calories: 370

Fat: 20g

Protein: 45g

Carbohydrates: 2g

383.   Monkey Salad

Preparation Time : 5 minutes Cooking Time : 7 minutes **Servings:** 1

Ingredients:

2 tbsp. butter

1 cup unsweetened coconut flakes

1 cup raw, unsalted cashews

1 cup raw, unsalted s

1 cup 90% dark chocolate shavings

Directions :

In a skillet, melt the butter on a medium heat.

Add the coconut flakes and sauté until lightly browned for 4 minutes.

Add the cashews and s and sauté for 3 minutes. Remove from the heat and sprinkle with dark chocolate shavings.

Serve!

Nutrition:

Calories: 320

Carbs: 5 g

Fat: 11 g

Protein: 6 g

Fiber: 4 g

Chapter 7:

Dessert Recipes

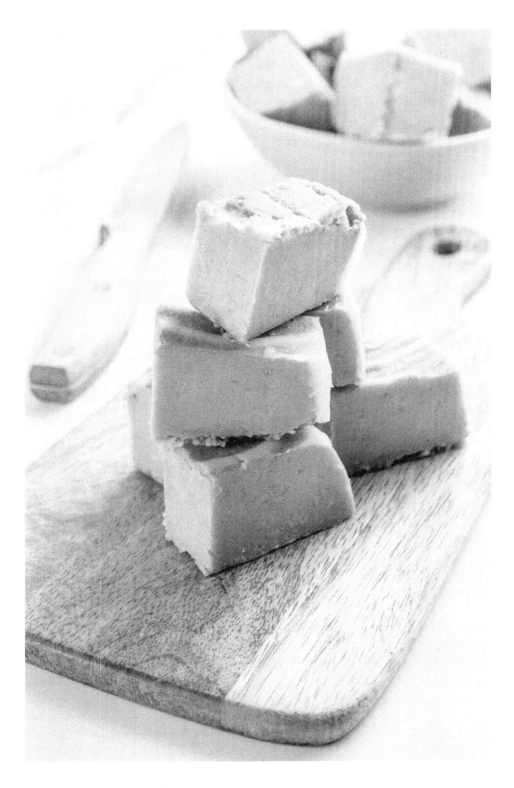

384. Bread Dough and Amaretto Dessert

Preparation Time: 15 Minutes
Cooking Time: 8 Minutes
Servings: 12
Ingredients:
1 lb. Bread dough
1 Cup sugar
½ Cup butter
1 Cup heavy cream
oz. Chocolate chips
2 Tbsp. amaretto liqueur
Directions:
Turn dough, cut into 20 slices and cut each piece in halves.
Put the dough pieces with spray sugar and butter, put this into the air fryer's basket, and cook them at 350°F for 5 minutes. Turn them, cook for 3 minutes still. Move to a platter.
Melt the heavy cream in a pan over medium heat, put chocolate chips and turn until they melt.
Put in liqueur, turn and move to a bowl.
Serve bread dippers with the sauce.
Nutrition:
Calories: 179
Total Fat: 18g
Total carbs: 17g

385. Bread Pudding

Preparation Time: 10 Minutes
Cooking Time: 10 Minutes
Servings: 4
Ingredients:
6 Glazed doughnuts
1 Cup cherries
4 Egg yolks
1 and ½ Cups whipping cream
½ Cup raisins
¼ Cup sugar
½ Cup chocolate chips
Directions:
Mix in cherries with whipping cream and egg in a bowl, then turn properly.
Mix in raisins with chocolate chips, sugar, and doughnuts in a bowl, then stir.
Combine the two mixtures, pour into an oiled pan, then into the air fryer, and cook at 310°F for 1 hour.
Cool pudding before cutting.

Serve.
Nutrition:
Calories: 456
Total Fat: 11g
Total carbs: 6g

386. Wrapped Pears

Preparation Time: 10 Minutes
Cooking Time: 10 Minutes
Servings: 4
Ingredients:
4 Puff pastry sheets
oz. Vanilla custard
2 Pears
1 Egg
½ Tbsp. cinnamon powder
2 Tbsp. sugar
Directions:
Put wisp pastry slices on a flat surface, add a spoonful of vanilla custard at the center of each, add pear halves and wrap.
Combine pears with egg, cinnamon, and spray sugar, put into the air fryer's basket, then cook at 320°F for 15 minutes.
Split portions on plates.
Serve.
Nutrition:
Calories: 285
Total Fat: 14g
Total carbs: 30g

387. Air Fried Bananas

Preparation Time: 5 Minutes
Cooking Time: 10 Minutes
Servings: 4
Ingredients:
3 Tbsp. butter
2 Eggs
8 Bananas
½ Cup corn flour
3 Tbsp. cinnamon sugar
1 Cup panko
Directions:
Heat a pan with the butter over medium heat, put panko, turn and cook for 4 minutes, then move to a bowl.
Dredge each in flour, panko, and egg mixture, place in the basket of the air fryer, gratinate with cinnamon sugar, and cook at 280°F for 10 minutes.

Serve immediately.
Nutrition:
Calories: 337
Total fat: 3g
Total carbs: 23g

388.   Tasty Banana Cake
Preparation Time: 10 Minutes
Cooking Time: 30 Minutes
Servings: 4
Ingredients:
1 Tbsp. butter, soft
1 Egg
1/3 Cup brown sugar
2 Tbsp. honey
1 Banana
1 Cup white flour
1 Tbsp. baking powder
½ Tbsp. cinnamon powder
Cooking spray
Directions:
Grease the cake pan with cooking spray.
Mix in butter with honey, sugar, banana, cinnamon, egg, flour, and baking powder in a bowl, then beat.
Put the mix in a cake pan with cooking spray, put into the air fryer, and cook at 350°F for 30 minutes.
Allow to cool, then slice it.
Serve.
Nutrition:
Calories: 435
Total Fat: 7g
Total carbs: 15g

389.   Peanut Butter Fudge
Preparation Time: 10 Minutes
Cooking Time: 10 Minutes
Servings: 20
Ingredients:
1/4 Cup almonds, toasted and chopped
12 oz. Smooth peanut butter
Drops liquid stevia
3 Tbsp. coconut oil
4 Tbsp. coconut cream
Pinch of salt
Directions:
Line a baking tray with parchment paper.
Melt coconut oil in a pan over low heat. Add peanut butter, coconut cream, stevia, and salt to a saucepan. Stir well.

Pour fudge mixture into the prepared baking tray and sprinkle chopped almonds on top.
Place the tray in the refrigerator for 1 hour or until set.
Slice and serve.
Nutrition:
Calories: 131
Fat: 12g
Carbs: 4g
Sugar: 2g
Protein: 5g
Cholesterol: 0mg

390.   Cocoa Cake
Preparation Time: 5 Minutes
Cooking Time: 17 Minutes
Servings: 6
Ingredients:
4 oz. Butter
3 Eggs
3 oz. Sugar
1 Tbsp. cocoa powder
3 oz. Flour
½ Tbsp. lemon juice
Directions:
Mix in 1 tablespoon butter with cocoa powder in a bowl and beat.
Mix in the rest of the butter with eggs, flour, sugar, and lemon juice in another bowl, blend properly and move the half into a cake pan
Put half of the cocoa blend, spread, add the rest of the butter layer, and crest with remaining cocoa.
Put into the air fryer and cook at 360° F for 17 minutes.
Allow it to cool before slicing.
Serve.
Nutrition:
Calories: 221
Total Fat: 5g
Total carbs: 12g

391.   Bounty Bars
Preparation Time: 20 Minutes
Cooking Time: 0 Minutes
Servings: 12
Ingredients:
1 Cup coconut cream
3 Cups shredded unsweetened coconut
1/4 Cup extra virgin coconut oil
½ Teaspoon vanilla powder

1/4 Cup powdered erythritol
1 ½ oz. Cocoa butter
5 oz. Dark chocolate

Directions:

Heat the oven at 350°F and toast the coconut in it for 5-6 minutes. Remove from the oven once toasted and set aside to cool.

Take a bowl of medium size and add coconut oil, coconut cream, vanilla, erythritol, and shredded coconut. Mix the ingredients well to prepare a smooth mixture.

Make 12 bars of equal size with the help of your hands from the prepared mixture and adjust in the tray lined with parchment paper.

Place the tray in the fridge for around one hour and, in the meantime, put the cocoa butter and dark chocolate in a glass bowl.

Heat a cup of water in a saucepan over medium heat and place the bowl over it to melt the cocoa butter and the dark chocolate.

Remove from the heat once melted properly, mix well until blended, and set it aside to cool.

Take the coconut bars and coat them with dark chocolate mixture one by one using a wooden stick. Adjust on the tray lined with parchment paper and drizzle the remaining mixture over them.

Refrigerate for around one hour before you serve the delicious bounty bars.

Nutrition:

Calories: 230
Fat: 25g
Carbohydrates: 5g
Protein: 32g

392.   Simple Cheesecake

Preparation Time: 10 Minutes
Cooking Time: 15 Minutes
Servings: 15
Ingredients:

1 lb. Cream cheese
½ Tbsp. vanilla extract
2 Eggs
4 Tbsp. sugar
1 Cup graham crackers
2 Tbsp. butter

Directions:

Mix in butter with crackers in a bowl.

Compress crackers blend to the bottom of a cake pan, put into the air fryer, and cook at 350°F for 4 minutes.

Mix cream cheese with sugar, vanilla, egg in a bowl and beat properly.

Sprinkle filling on crackers crust and cook the cheesecake in the air fryer at 310°F for 15 minutes.

Keep the cake in the fridge for 3 hours, slice.

Serve.

Nutrition:

Calories: 257
Total Fat: 18g
Total carbs: 22g

393.   Chocolate Almond Butter Brownie

Preparation Time: 10 Minutes
Cooking Time: 16 Minutes
Servings: 4
Ingredients:

1 Cup bananas, overripe
½ Cup almond butter, melted
1 Scoop protein powder
2 Tbsp. unsweetened cocoa powder

Directions:

Preheat the air fryer to 325°F. Grease the air fryer baking pan and set it aside.

Blend all ingredients in a blender until smooth.

Pour the batter into the prepared pan and place it in the air fryer basket to cook for 16 minutes.

Serve and enjoy.

Nutrition:

Calories: 82
Fat: 2g
Carbs: 11g
Sugar: 5g
Protein: 7g
Cholesterol: 16mg

394.   Almond Butter Fudge

Preparation Time: 10 Minutes
Cooking Time: 10 Minutes
Servings: 18
Ingredients:

3/4 Cup creamy almond butter
1 ½ Cups unsweetened chocolate chips

Directions:

Line 8x4-inch pan with parchment paper and set aside.

Add chocolate chips and almond butter into the double boiler and cook over medium heat until the chocolate-butter mixture is melted. Stir well.

Place the mixture into the prepared pan and place in the freezer until set.

Slice and serve.

Nutrition:
Calories: 197
Fat: 16g
Carbs: 7g
Sugar: 1g
Protein: 4g
Cholesterol: 0mg

395.   Apple Bread

Preparation Time: 5 Minutes
Cooking Time: 40 Minutes
Servings: 6
Ingredients:
3 Cups apples
1 Cup sugar
1 Tbsp. vanilla
2 Eggs
1 Tbsp. apple pie spice
2 Cups white flour
1 Tbsp. baking powder
1 Butter stick
1 Cup water
Directions:
Mix the eggs with one butter stick, sugar, vanilla, and apple pie spice, then turn using a mixer.
Put apples and turn properly.
Mix baking powder with flour in another bowl and turn.
Blend the two mixtures, turn and move it to a springform pan.
Put the pan into the air fryer and cook at 320°F for 40 minutes
Slice.
Serve.
Nutrition:
Calories: 401
Total Fat: 9g
Total carbs: 29g

396.   Banana Bread

Preparation Time: 5 Minutes
Cooking Time: 40 Minutes
Servings: 6
Ingredients:
¾ Cup sugar
1/3 Cup butter
1 Tbsp. vanilla extract
1 Egg
2 Bananas

1 Tbsp. baking powder
1 and ½ Cups flour
½ Tbsp. baking soda
1/3 Cup milk
1 and ½ Tbsp. cream of tartar
Cooking spray
Directions:
Mix the milk with cream of tartar, vanilla, egg, sugar, bananas, and butter in a bowl, then mix all.
Mix in flour with baking soda and baking powder.
Blend the two mixtures, turn properly, move into an oiled pan with cooking spray, put into the air fryer, and cook at 320°F for 40 minutes. Remove the bread, allow to cool, slice. Serve.
Nutrition:
Calories: 540 Total Fat: 16g Total carbs: 28g

397.   Mini Lava Cakes

Preparation Time: 5 Minutes
Cooking Time: 20 Minutes
Servings: 3
Ingredients:
1 Egg
4 Tbsp. sugar
2 Tbsp. olive oil
4 Tbsp. milk
4 Tbsp. flour
1 Tbsp. cocoa powder
½ Tbsp. baking powder
½ Tbsp. orange zest
A pinch of salt
Directions:
Mix in egg with sugar, flour, salt, oil, milk, orange zest, baking powder, and cocoa powder, turn properly. Move it to oiled ramekins.
Put ramekins in the air fryer and cook at 320°F for 20 minutes.
Serve warm.
Nutrition:
Calories: 329
Total Fat: 8.5g
Total carbs: 12.4g

398.   Ricotta Ramekins

Preparation Time: 10 Minutes
Cooking Time: 1 Hour
Servings: 4
Ingredients:
6 Eggs, whisked
1 and ½ Pounds ricotta cheese, soft

½ Pound stevia
1 Teaspoon vanilla extract
½ Teaspoon baking powder
Cooking spray
Directions:
In a bowl, mix the eggs with the ricotta and the other ingredients except for the cooking spray and whisk well.
Grease 4 ramekins with the cooking spray, pour the ricotta cream in each and bake at 360 degrees F for 1 hour.
Serve cold.
Nutrition:
Calories: 180
Fat: 5.3
Fiber: 5.4
Carbs: 11.5
Protein: 4

399. Strawberry Sorbet

Preparation Time: 15 Minutes
Cooking Time: 10 Minutes
Servings: 6
Ingredients:
1 Cup strawberries, chopped
1 Tablespoon of liquid honey
2 Tablespoons water
1 Tablespoon lemon juice
Directions:
Preheat the water and liquid honey until you get a homogenous liquid.
Blend the strawberries until smooth and combine them with the honey liquid and lemon juice.
Transfer the strawberry mixture to the ice cream maker and churn it for 20 minutes or until the sorbet is thick.
Scoop the cooked sorbet in the ice cream cups.
Nutrition:
Calories: 30
Fat: 0.4g
Fiber: 1.4g
Carbs: 14.9g
Protein: 0.9g

400. Crispy Apples

Preparation Time: 10 Minutes
Cooking Time: 10 Minutes
Servings: 4
Ingredients:
2 Tbsp. cinnamon powder

5 Apples
½ Tbsp. nutmeg powder
1 Tbsp. maple syrup
½ Cup water
4 Tbsp. butter
¼ Cup flour
¾ Cup oats
¼ Cup brown sugar
Directions:
Get the apples in a pan, put in nutmeg, maple syrup, cinnamon, and water.
Mix in butter with flour, sugar, salt, and oat, turn, put a spoonful of the blend over apples, get into the air fryer and cook at 350°F for 10 minutes.
Serve while warm.
Nutrition:
Calories: 387
Total Fat: 5.6g
Total carbs: 12.4g

401. Cocoa Cookies

Preparation Time: 10 Minutes
Cooking Time: 14 Minutes
Servings: 12
Ingredients:
6 oz. Coconut oil
6 Eggs
3 oz. Cocoa powder
2 Tbsp. vanilla
½ Tbsp. baking powder
4 oz. Cream cheese
5 Tbsp. sugar
Directions:
Mix the eggs with sugar, coconut oil, baking powder, cocoa powder, cream cheese, vanilla in a blender, then sway and turn using a mixer.
Get it into a lined baking dish and put it into the fryer at 320°F, and bake for 14 minutes.
Split cookie sheet into rectangles.
Serve.
Nutrition:
Calories: 149 Total Fat: 2.4g Total carbs: 27.2g

402. Cinnamon Pears

Preparation Time: 2 Hours
Cooking Time: 0 Minutes
Servings: 6
Ingredients:
2 Pears
1 Teaspoon ground cinnamon

1 Tablespoon Erythritol
1 Teaspoon liquid stevia
4 Teaspoons butter
Directions:
Cut the pears on the halves.
Then scoop the seeds from the pears with the help of the scooper.
In a shallow bowl, mix up together Erythritol and ground cinnamon.
Sprinkle every pear half with cinnamon mixture and drizzle with liquid stevia.
Then add butter and wrap in the foil.
Bake the pears for 25 minutes at 365°F.
Then remove the pears from the foil and transfer them to the serving plates.
Nutrition:
Calories: 96
Fat: 4.4g
Fiber: 1.4g Carbs: 3.9g
Protein: 0.9g

403.   Cherry Compote
Preparation Time: 2 Hours
Cooking Time: 0 Minutes
Servings: 6
Ingredients:
2 Peaches, pitted, halved
1 Cup cherries, pitted
½ Cup grape juice
½ Cup strawberries
1 Tablespoon liquid honey
1 Teaspoon vanilla extract
1 Teaspoon ground cinnamon
Directions:
Pour grape juice into the saucepan.
Add vanilla extract and ground cinnamon. Bring the liquid to a boil.
After this, put peaches, cherries, and strawberries in the hot grape juice and bring them to a boil.
Remove the mixture from heat, add liquid honey, and close the lid.
Let the compote rest for 20 minutes.
Carefully mix up the compote and transfer it to the serving plate.
Nutrition:
Calories: 80
Fat: 0.4g
Fiber: 2.4g
Carbs: 19.9g
Protein: 0.9g

404.   Vanilla Apple Pie
Preparation Time: 15 Minutes
Cooking Time: 50 Minutes
Servings: 8
Ingredients:
3 Apples, sliced
½ Teaspoon ground cinnamon
1 Teaspoon vanilla extract
1 Tablespoon Erythritol
7 oz. Yeast roll dough
1 Egg, beaten
Directions:
Roll up the dough and cut it into two parts.
Line a springform pan with baking paper.
Place the first dough part in the springform pan.
Then arrange the apples over the dough and sprinkle it with Erythritol, vanilla extract, and ground cinnamon.
Then cover the apples with the remaining dough and secure the edges of the pie with the help of the fork.
Make the small cuts on the surface of the pie.
Brush the pie with the beaten egg and bake it for 50 minutes at 375F.
Cool the cooked pie well, and then remove it from the springform pan.
Cut it on the servings.
Nutrition:
Calories: 140
Fat: 3.4g
Fiber: 3.4g
Carbs: 23.9g
Protein: 2.9g

405.   Creamy Strawberries
Preparation Time: 15 Minutes
Cooking Time: 10 Minutes
Servings: 6
Ingredients:
6 Tablespoons almond butter
1 Tablespoon Erythritol
1 Cup milk
1 Teaspoon vanilla extract
1 Cup strawberries, sliced
Directions:
Pour milk into a saucepan.
Add Erythritol, vanilla extract, and almond butter.
With the help of a hand mixer, mix up the liquid until smooth and bring it to a boil.
Then remove the mixture from the heat and let it cool.

The cooled mixture will be thick.

Put the strawberries in serving glasses and top with the thick almond butter dip.

Nutrition:
Calories: 192
Fat: 14.4g
Fiber: 3.4g
Carbs: 10.9g
Protein: 1.9g

406. Special Brownies

Preparation Time: 10 Minutes
Cooking Time: 22 Minutes
Servings: 4
Ingredients:
1 Egg
1/3 Cup cocoa powder
1/3 Cup sugar
7 Tbsp. butter
½ Tbsp. vanilla extract
¼ Cup white flour
¼ Cup walnuts
½ Tbsp. baking powder
1 Tbsp. peanut butter
A pinch of salt
Directions:
Warm pan with six butter tablespoons and the sugar over medium heat, turn, cook for 5 minutes, move to a bowl, put salt, egg, cocoa powder, vanilla extract, walnuts, baking powder, and flour, turn mix properly and into a pan.

Mix peanut butter with one butter tablespoon in a bowl, heat in the microwave for some seconds, turn properly, and sprinkle brownies blend over.

Put in the air fryer and bake at 320° F for 17 minutes. Allow brownies to cool, cut.

Serve.

Nutrition:
Calories: 438
Total Fat: 18g
Total carbs: 16.5g

407. Apple Couscous Pudding

Preparation Time: 10 Minutes
Cooking Time: 25 Minutes
Servings: 4
Ingredients:
½ Cup couscous
1 and ½ Cups milk
¼ Cup apple, cored and chopped

3 Tablespoons stevia
½ Teaspoon rose water
1 Tablespoon orange zest, grated
Directions:
Heat up a pan with the milk over medium heat, Add the couscous and the rest of the ingredients, whisk, simmer for 25 minutes, divide into bowls and serve.

Nutrition:
Calories: 150
Fat: 4.5
Fiber: 5.5
Carbs: 7.5
Protein: 4

408. Blueberry Scones

Preparation Time: 10 Minutes
Cooking Time: 10 Minutes
Servings: 10
Ingredients:
1 Cup white flour
1 Cup blueberries
2 Eggs
½ Cup heavy cream
½ Cup butter
5 Tbsp. sugar
2 Tbsp. vanilla extract
2 Tbsp. baking powder
A pinch of salt
Directions:
Mix in flour, baking powder, salt, and blueberries in a bowl, then turn.

Mix heavy cream with vanilla extract, sugar, butter, and eggs and turn properly.

Blend the two mixtures, squeeze till the dough is ready, obtain ten triangles from the mix, put on a baking sheet into the air fryer, and cook them at 320°F for 10 minutes.

Serve cold.

Nutrition:
Calories: 525
Total Fat: 21g
Total carbs: 37g

409. Papaya Cream

Preparation Time: 10 Minutes
Cooking Time: 0 Minutes
Servings: 2
Ingredients:
1 Cup papaya, peeled and chopped

1 Cup heavy cream
1 Tablespoon stevia
½ Teaspoon vanilla extract
Directions:
In a blender, combine the cream with the papaya and the other ingredients, pulse well, divide into cups and serve cold.
Nutrition:
Calories: 182
Fat: 3.1
Fiber: 2.3
Carbs: 3.5
Protein: 2

410. Ginger Cheesecake

Preparation Time: 20 Minutes
Cooking Time: 20 Minutes
Servings: 6
Ingredients:
2 Tbsp. butter
½ Cup ginger cookies
oz. Cream cheese
2 Eggs
½ Cup sugar
1 Tbsp. rum
½ Tbsp. vanilla extract
½ Tbsp. nutmeg
Directions:
Spread a pan with the butter and sprinkle cookie crumbs on the bottom.
Whisk cream cheese with sugar, rum, vanilla, nutmeg, and eggs, beat properly, and sprinkle the cookie crumbs.
Put in the air fryer and cook at 340°F for 20 minutes.
Allow the cheesecake to cool in the fridge for 2 hours before slicing.
Serve.
Nutrition:
Calories: 312
Total Fat: 9.8g
Total carbs: 18g

411. Almonds and Oats Pudding

Preparation Time: 10 Minutes
Cooking Time: 15 Minutes
Servings: 4
Ingredients:
1 Tablespoon lemon juice
The zest of 1 lime
1 and ½ Cups almond milk

1 Teaspoon almond extract
½ Cup oats
2 Tablespoons stevia
½ Cup silver almonds, chopped
Directions:
In a pan, combine the almond milk with the lime zest and the other ingredients, whisk, bring to a simmer and cook over medium heat for 15 minutes.
Divide the mix into bowls and serve cold.
Nutrition:
Calories: 174
Fat: 12.1
Fiber: 3.2
Carbs: 3.9
Protein: 4.8

.

Chapter 8:

Morning Snacks

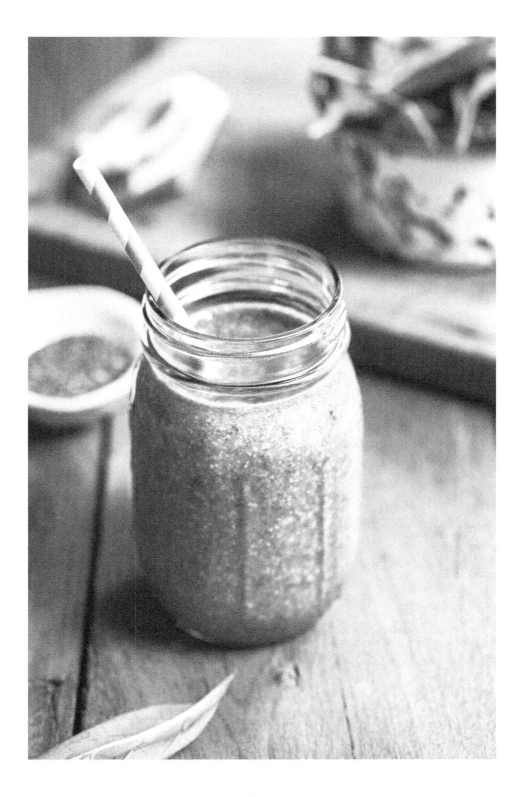

412. Sweet Green Smoothie

Preparation Time: 10 minutes
Cooking Time: 0 minutes
Servings: 1
Ingredients:
2 tablespoons flax seeds
½ cup wheatgrass
1 mango
1 cup pomegranate juice
Directions:
Add all ingredients to the blender and blend until smooth and creamy.
Serve immediately and enjoy.
Nutrition: Calories: 177, Fat: 1, Carbs: 21, Protein: 5

413. Avocado Mango Smoothie

Preparation Time: 10 minutes
Cooking Time: 0 minutes
Servings: 2
Ingredients:
1 cup ice cubes
½ cup mango
½ avocado
1 tablespoon ginger
3 kale leaves
1 cup coconut water
Directions:
Toss all your ingredients into your blender, then process until smooth.
Serve and Enjoy.
Nutrition: Calories: 290, Fat: 3, Carbs: 18, Protein: 11

414. Super Healthy Green Smoothie

Preparation Time: 10 minutes
Cooking Time: 0 minutes
Servings: 2
Ingredients:
1 teaspoon spirulina powder
1 cup coconut water
2 cups mixed greens
1 tablespoon ginger
4 tablespoon lemon juice
2 celery stalks
1 cup cucumber, chopped
1 green pear, core removed
1 banana

Directions:
Add all ingredients to the blender and blend until smooth and creamy.
2. Serve immediately and enjoy.
Nutrition: Calories: 161, Fat: 1, Carbs: 19, Protein: 7

415. Spinach Coconut Smoothie

Preparation Time: 10 minutes
Cooking Time: 0 minutes
Servings: 2
Ingredients:
2 tablespoons unsweetened coconut flakes
2 cups fresh pineapple
½ cup coconut water
1 ½ cups coconut milk
2 cups fresh spinach
Directions:
Add all ingredients to the blender and blend until smooth and creamy.
Serve immediately and enjoy.
Nutrition: Calories: 290, Fat: 1, Carbs: 22, Protein: 8

416. Green Mango Smoothie

Preparation Time: 5 minutes
Cooking Time: 0 minutes
Servings: 1
Ingredients:
2 cups Spinach
1-2 cups Coconut Water
2 Mangos, Ripe, Peeled & Diced

Directions:
Blend everything together until smooth.
Nutrition: Calories: 120, Fat: 1, Carbs: 5, Protein: 8

417. Chia Seed Smoothie

Preparation Time: 5 minutes
Cooking Time: 0 minutes
Servings: 3
Ingredients:
¼ teaspoon Cinnamon
1 tablespoon Ginger, Fresh & Grated
Pinch Cardamom
1 tablespoon Chia Seeds
2 Medjool Dates, Pitted
1 cup Alfalfa Sprouts
1 cup Water
1 Banana

½ cup Coconut Milk, Unsweetened
Directions:
Blend everything together until smooth.
Nutrition: Calories: 412 Protein: 18.9g Carbs: 43.8gFat: 24.8g

418.   Mango Smoothie
Preparation Time: 5 minutes
Cooking Time: 0 minutes
Servings: 3
Ingredients:
1 Carrot, Peeled & Chopped
1 cup Strawberries
1 cup Water
1 cup Peaches, Chopped
1 Banana, Frozen & sliced
1 cup Mango, Chopped
Directions:
Blend everything together until smooth.
Nutrition: Calories: 221, Fat: 1, Carbs: 5, Protein: 4

419.   Spinach Peach Banana Smoothie
Preparation Time: 10 minutes
Cooking Time: 0 minutes
Servings: 2
Ingredients:
1 cup baby spinach
2 cups coconut water
1 tablespoon agave syrup
2 ripe bananas
2 ripe peaches, pitted and chopped
Directions:
Add all ingredients to the blender and blend until smooth and creamy.
Serve immediately and enjoy.
Nutrition: Calories: 163, Fat: 1, Carbs: 4, Protein: 6

420.   Salty Green Smoothie
Preparation Time: 10 minutes
Cooking Time: 0 minutes
Servings: 2
Ingredients:
1 cup ice cubes
¼ tablespoon liquid aminos
1 ½ tablespoon sea salt
2 limes, peeled and quartered
1 avocado, pitted and peeled
1 cup kale leaves
1 cucumber, chopped

2 cups tomato, chopped
¼ cup water
Directions:
Add all ingredients to the blender and blend until smooth and creamy.
Serve immediately and enjoy.
Nutrition: Calories: 108, Fat: 1, Carbs: 1, Protein: 4

421.   Watermelon Strawberry Smoothie
Preparation Time: 10 minutes
Cooking Time: 0 minutes
Servings: 2
Ingredients:
1 cup coconut milk yogurt
½ cup strawberries
2 cups fresh watermelon
1 banana
Directions:
Toss all your ingredients into your blender, then process until smooth.
Serve and Enjoy.
Nutrition: Calories: 160, fat 1, carbs 3, protein 4

422.   Watermelon Kale Smoothie
Preparation Time: 10 minutes
Cooking Time: 0 minutes
Servings: 2
Ingredients:
8 ounce water
1 orange, peeled
3 cups kale, chopped
1 banana, peeled
2 cups watermelon, chopped
1 celery, chopped
Directions:
Add all ingredients to the blender and blend until smooth and creamy.
Serve immediately and Enjoy.
Nutrition: Calories: 122, Fat: 1, Carbs: 5, Protein: 1

423.   Mix Berry Watermelon Smoothie
Preparation Time: 10 minutes
Cooking Time: 0 minutes
Servings: 2
Ingredients:
1 cup alkaline water
2 fresh lemon juices
¼ cup fresh mint leaves

1 ½ cup mixed berries

2 cups watermelon

Directions:

Toss all your ingredients into your blender, then process until smooth. Serve immediately and Enjoy.

Nutrition: Calories: 188, Fat: 1, Carbs: 2, Protein: 1

424. Healthy Green Smoothie

Preparation Time: 10 minutes

Cooking Time: 0 minutes

Servings: 3

Ingredients:

1 cup water

1 fresh lemon, peeled

1 avocado

1 cucumber, peeled

1 cup spinach

1 cup ice cubes

Directions:

Add all ingredients to the blender and blend until smooth and creamy.

Serve immediately and enjoy.

Nutrition: Calories: 160, Fat: 13, Carbs: 12, Protein: 2

425. Apple Spinach Cucumber Smoothie

Preparation Time: 10 minutes

Cooking Time: 0 minutes

Servings: 1

Ingredients:

¾ cup water

½ green apple, diced

¾ cup spinach

½ cucumber

Directions:

Add all ingredients to the blender and blend until smooth and creamy.

Serve immediately and enjoy.

Nutrition: Calories: 90, Fat: 1, Carbs: 21, Protein: 1

426. Refreshing Lime Smoothie

Preparation Time: 10 minutes

Cooking Time: 0 minutes

Servings: 2

Ingredients:

1 cup ice cubes

20 drops liquid stevia

2 fresh lime, peeled and halved

1 tablespoon lime zest, grated

½ cucumber, chopped

1 avocado, pitted and peeled

2 cups spinach

1 tablespoon creamed coconut

¾ cup coconut water

Directions:

Add all ingredients to the blender and blend until smooth and creamy.

Serve immediately and enjoy.

Nutrition: Calories: 312, Fat: 3, Carbs: 28, Protein: 4

427. Broccoli Green Smoothie

Preparation Time: 10 minutes

Cooking Time: 0 minutes

Servings: 2

Ingredients:

1 celery, peeled and chopped

1 lemon, peeled

1 apple, diced

1 banana

1 cup spinach

1/2 cup broccoli

Directions:

Add all ingredients to the blender and blend until smooth and creamy.

Serve immediately and enjoy.

Nutrition: Calories: 121, Fat: 1, Carbs: 18, Protein: 1

428. Spiced Popcorn

Preparation Time: 5 minutes

Cooking Time: 5 minutes

Servings: 4

Ingredients:

3 tablespoons olive oil

½ cup popcorn kernels

Cooking spray

1 teaspoon garlic powder

1 teaspoon onion powder

½ teaspoon smoked paprika

½ teaspoon salt

1/8 teaspoon cayenne pepper

Directions:

Heat the olive oil in the pot. Add 3 popcorn kernels, and when one of the kernels pops, add the rest. Cover and shake well until fully popped, transfer the popcorn to a large bowl.

Spray the popcorn with cooking spray. Use clean hands to toss the popcorn, mixing it thoroughly. In

a small bowl, mix together the garlic powder, onion powder, paprika, salt and cayenne. Add some spice mix of your taste and toss until coated.
Nutrition: Calories: 210, Fat: 17, Carbs: 3, Protein: 16

429. Baked Spinach Chips

Preparation Time: 5 minutes
Cooking Time: 15 minutes
Servings: 4
Ingredients:
Cooking spray
5 ounces baby spinach, washed and patted dry
2 tablespoons olive oil
1 teaspoon garlic powder
½ teaspoon salt
1/8 teaspoon freshly ground black pepper
Directions:
Preheat the oven to 350°F. Coat 2 baking sheets with cooking spray. Place the spinach in a large bowl. Mix in olive oil, garlic powder, salt, and pepper, and toss until evenly coated.
Spread the spinach in a single layer on the baking sheets. Bake until the spinach leaves are crispy and slightly browned. Store spinach chips in a resealable container at room temperature for up to 1 week.
Nutrition: Calories: 451, Fat: 18, Carbs: 7, Protein: 12

430. Peanut Butter Yogurt Dip with Fruit

Preparation Time: 10 minutes
Cooking Time: 5 minutes
Servings: 4
Ingredients:
1 cup nonfat vanilla Greek yogurt
2 tablespoons natural creamy peanut butter
2 teaspoons honey
1 pear, cored and sliced
1 apple, cored and sliced
1 banana, sliced
Directions:
Whisk together the yogurt, peanut butter, and honey in a bowl. Serve the dip with the fruit on the side.
Nutrition: Calories: 421, Fat: 5, Carbs: 3, Protein: 10

431. Snickerdoodle Pecans

Preparation Time: 10 minutes
Cooking Time: 15 minutes
Servings: 8
Ingredients:
Cooking spray
1½ cups raw pecans
2 tablespoons brown sugar
2 tablespoons 100% maple syrup
½ teaspoon ground cinnamon
½ teaspoon vanilla extract
1/8 teaspoon salt
Directions:
Line and set the oven to 350°F. In a medium bowl, place the pecans. Add the brown sugar, maple syrup, cinnamon, vanilla and salt, tossing to evenly coat.
Place pecans in a single layer. Bake for about 12 minutes, until pecans are lightly browned and fragrant. Remove and let it cool for 10 minutes.
Nutrition: Calories: 321, Fat: 28, Carbs: 7, Protein: 42

432. Crispy Rye Bread Snacks with Guacamole and Anchovies

Preparation Time: 10 minutes
Cooking Time: 10 minutes
Servings: 4
Ingredients:
4 slices of rye bread
Guacamole
Anchovies in oil
Directions:
Cut each slice of bread into 3 strips of bread.
Place in the basket of the air fryer, without piling up, and we go in batches giving it the touch you want to give it. You can select 1800C, 10 minutes.
When you have all the crusty rye bread strips, put a layer of guacamole on top, whether homemade or commercial.
In each bread, place 2 anchovies on the guacamole.
Nutrition: Calories: 180Carbs: 4 g Fat: 11 g Protein: 4 g Fiber: 09 g

433. Mushrooms Stuffed with Tomato

Preparation Time: 5 minutes
Cooking Time: 50 minutes
Servings: 4
Ingredients:
8 large mushrooms
250g of minced meat
4 cloves of garlic
Extra virgin olive oil
Salt
Ground pepper
Flour, beaten egg and breadcrumbs
Frying oil
Fried Tomato Sauce
Directions:
Remove the stem from the mushrooms and chop it. Peel the garlic and chop. Put some extra virgin olive oil in a pan and add the garlic and mushroom stems. Sauté and add the minced meat. Sauté well until the meat is well cooked and season.
Fill the mushrooms with the minced meat.
Press well and take the freezer for 30 minutes.
Pass the mushrooms with flour, beaten egg and breadcrumbs. Beaten egg and breadcrumbs.
Place the mushrooms in the basket of the air fryer.
Select 20 minutes, 1800C.
Distribute the mushrooms once cooked in the dishes. Heat the tomato sauce and cover the stuffed mushrooms.
Nutrition: Calories: 160 Carbs: 2 g Fat: 11 g Protein: 4 g Fiber: 0 g

434. Fennel and Arugula Salad With Fig Vinaigrette

Preparation Time: 15 minutes
Cooking Time: 10 minutes
Servings: 6
Ingredients:
5 Ounces of washed and dried arugula
1 small fennel bulb, it can be either shaved or tiny sliced.
2 tablespoons of extra virgin oil or any cooking oil
1 teaspoon of lemon zest
1/2 teaspoon of salt
Pepper (freshly ground)
Pecorino
Directions:
Mix the arugula and shaved funnel in a serving bowl.

On another bowl, mix the olive oil or cooking oil, lemon zest, salt and pepper
Shake together until it becomes creamy and smooth.
Pour and dress over the salad, tossing gently for it to combine.
Peel or shave out some slices of pecorino and put it on top of the salad
Serve immediately
Nutrition: Protein: 2.1 gCarbohydrates: 14.3 gDietary Fiber: 3.4 gSugars: 9.1 gFat: 9.7 g

435. Mixed Potato Gratin

Preparation Time: 20 minutes
Cooking Time: 7 to 9 hours
Servings: 8
Ingredients:
6 Yukon Gold potatoes, thinly sliced
3 sweet potatoes, peeled and thinly sliced
2 onions, thinly sliced
4 garlic cloves, minced
3 tablespoons whole-wheat flour
4 cups 2% milk, divided
11/2 cups Roasted Vegetable Broth
3 tablespoons melted butter
1 teaspoon dried thyme leaves
11/2 cups shredded Havarti cheese
Directions:
Grease a 6-quart slow cooker with straight vegetable oil.
In the slow cooker, layer the potatoes, onions, and garlic.
In a large bowl, mix the flour with 1/2 cup of the milk until well combined.
Gradually add the remaining milk, stirring with a wire whisk to avoid lumps.
Stir in the vegetable broth, melted butter, and thyme leaves.
Pour the milk mixture over the potatoes in the slow cooker and top with the cheese.
Cover and cook on low for 7 to 9 hours, or until the potatoes are tender when pierced with a fork.
Nutrition: Calories: 415 CalCarbohydrates: 42 gSugar: 10 gFiber: 3 gFat: 22 gSaturated Fat: 13 gProtein: 17 gSodium: 431 mg

436.   Green Pea Guacamole

Preparation Time: 15 minutes
Cooking Time: 35 minutes
Servings: 4
Ingredients:
1 teaspoon of crushed garlic
1 chopped tomato
3 cups of frozen green peas (chopped)
5 Green chopped onions
1/6 teaspoon of hot sauce
1/2 teaspoon of grounded cumin
1/2 cup of lime juice
Directions:
Blend the peas, garlic, lime juice and cumin until it is smoothened
Stir in the tomatoes, green onion and hot sauce into the mixture
Then add salt to taste
Cover it and put into the refrigerator for a minimum of 30 minutes.
This will allow the flavor to blend very well.
Nutrition:
Calories: 40.7, CalFat: 0.2 g, Cholesterol: 0.0 mg, Sodium: 157.4 mg, Carbohydrates: 7.6 g, Dietary Fiber: 1.7 g, Protein: 2.7 g

Chapter 9:

Afternoon Snacks

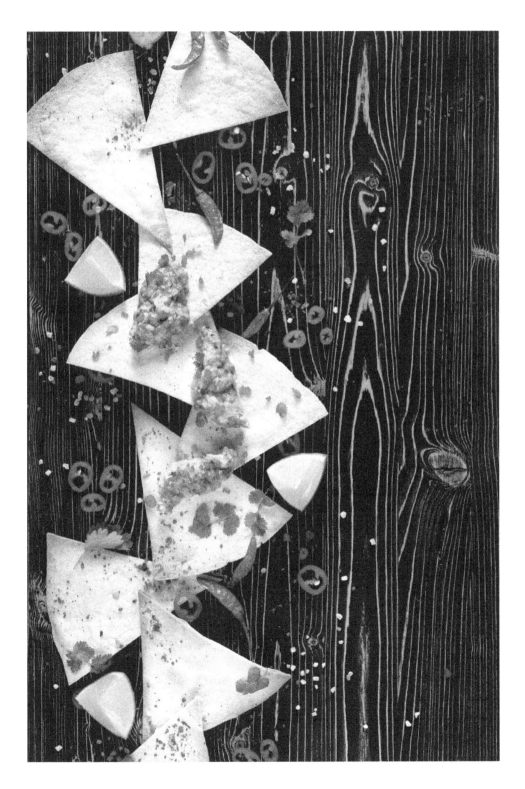

437. Almond-Stuffed Dates

Preparation Time: 5 minutes
Cooking Time: 3 minutes
Servings: 4
Ingredients:
20 raw almonds
20 pitted dates
Directions:
Stuffed one almond into each of 20 dates. Serve at room temperature.
Nutrition: Calories: 223, Fat: 12, Carbs: 4, Protein: 12

438. Peanut Butter Chocolate Chip Energy Bites

Preparation Time: 35 minutes
Cooking Time: 5 minutes
Servings: 12
Ingredients:
1 cup gluten-free old-fashioned oats
¾ cup natural creamy peanut butter
½ cup unsweetened coconut flakes
½ teaspoon vanilla extract
2 tablespoons honey
¼ cup dark chocolate chips
Directions:
Line the sheet and preheat the oven to 350°F. Spread the oats. Bake until the oats are browned. Let it cool. Blend the oats, peanut butter, coconut, vanilla, and honey until smooth. Transfer the batter into a medium bowl, and fold in the chocolate chips. Spoon out a tablespoon of batter. Use clean hands to roll into a 2-inch ball and place it on the baking sheet. Repeat for the remaining batter, making a total of 12 balls. Let it chill to set.
Nutrition: Calories: 333, Fat: 18, Carbs: 7, Protein: 12

439. No-Cook Pistachio-Cranberry Quinoa Bites

Preparation Time: 30 minutes
Cooking Time: 0 minutes
Servings: 12
Ingredients:
½ cup quinoa
¾ cup natural almond butter
¾ cup gluten-free old-fashioned oats
2 tablespoons honey
1/8 teaspoon salt
¼ cup unsalted shelled pistachios, roughly chopped
¼ cup dried cranberries
Directions:
Blend the quinoa until it turns into a flour consistency. Mix in almond butter, oats, honey and salt, and blend until smooth.
Transfer into a medium bowl, and gently fold in the pistachios and cranberries. Spoon out a tablespoon of the batter. Use clean hands to roll into a 2-inch ball and place it into a container. Repeat for the remaining batter, making a total of 12 balls. Let it chill to set.
Nutrition: Calories: 214, Fat: 19, Carbs: 3, Protein: 21

440. No-Bake Honey-Almond Granola Bars

Preparation Time: 15 minutes, plus 1 to 2 hours to chill
Cooking Time: 0 minutes
Servings: 8
Ingredients:
Cooking spray
1 cup pitted dates
¼ cup honey
¾ cup natural creamy almond butter
¾ cup gluten-free rolled oats
2 tablespoons raw almonds, chopped
2 tablespoons pumpkin seeds
Directions:
Line an 8-by-8-inch baking dish with parchment paper, and coat the paper with cooking spray. In a food processor or blender, add the dates and blend until they reach a paste-like consistency. Add the honey, almond butter and oats, and blend until well combined. Transfer the mixture to a medium bowl. Mix almonds and pumpkin seeds, and gently fold until well combined. Spoon the mixture into the prepared baking dish. Spread the mixture evenly, using clean fingers to push down the mixture, so it is compact. Let it chill for at least 1 to 2 hours.
Remove from the refrigerator and cut into 8 bars. Carefully remove each bar from the baking dish and wrap it individually in plastic wrap. Place bars in the refrigerator until ready to grab and go.
Nutrition: Calories: 121, Fat: 1, Carbs: 8, Protein: 12

441. Cottage Cheese-Filled Avocado

Preparation Time: 5 minutes
Cooking Time: 3 minutes
Servings: 4
Ingredients:
½ cup low-fat cottage cheese
¼ cup cherry tomatoes, quartered
2 avocados, halved and pitted
4 teaspoons pumpkin seeds
¼ teaspoon salt
1/8 teaspoon freshly ground black pepper
Directions:
Mix together the cottage cheese and tomatoes in a bowl. Spoon 2 tablespoons of the cheese-tomato mixture onto each of the avocado halves. Top each with 1 teaspoon of pumpkin seeds, and sprinkle with salt and pepper.
Nutrition: Calories: 212, Fat: 15, Carbs: 3, Protein: 18

442. Toast with Balsamic Glaze

Preparation Time: 5 minutes
Cooking Time: 10 minutes
Servings: 2
Ingredients:
1 tablespoon brown sugar
5 cherry tomatoes, halved
1/8 teaspoon salt
½ cup Vinegar
½ loaf Bread
1/8 teaspoon freshly ground black pepper
Directions:
Mix vinegar and brown sugar in a hot saucepan, continue stirring until it dissolves. Bring the mixture and simmer until the vinegar is reduced by half and thickens. Let it cool for 10 minutes.
Take out the flesh and mash it into the toasted bread. Top it with tomatoes and season. Then, add the balsamic glaze to each toast.
Nutrition: Calories: 214, fat 8, carbs 4, protein 10

443. Whole-Wheat Chocolate-Banana Quesadillas

Preparation Time: 5 minutes
Cooking Time: 5 minutes
Servings: 4
Ingredients:
Cooking spray
2 (10-inch) whole-wheat tortillas
1 ½ ounce 60% dark chocolate
2 tablespoons natural creamy peanut butter
1 medium banana, thinly sliced
Directions:
Add a tortilla and warm for 30 seconds on each side in a pan. Melt the chocolate in the microwave, about 1 minute, stirring halfway through. Using a spatula, spread the peanut butter onto 1 tortilla to the edges. Top with the banana slices, and drizzle the chocolate over the peanut butter.
Topped with the second tortilla, pressing down gently with the palm of your hand. Cut into 8 pieces and serve.
Nutrition: Calories: 212, Fat: 5, Carbs: 3, Protein: 10

444. Whole-Grain Mexican-Style Rollups

Preparation Time: 3 hours and 10 minutes
Cooking Time: 3 minutes
Servings: 4
Ingredients:
½ cup nonfat plain non-dairy Greek yogurt
½ cup non-dairy sour cream
¼ teaspoon salt
1 1/8 teaspoon freshly ground black pepper
1 cup shredded non-dairy cheese
1 15 ounces can low-sodium black beans
2 10-inch whole-wheat tortillas
Directions:
Mix together the yogurt, sour cream, salt, and pepper. Stir in the cheese and mashed beans. Lay the tortillas side by side on a cutting board. Spread 1 cup of the mixture onto each tortilla out to the edges.
Roll up each tortilla and cut off the uneven ends. Wrap each in plastic wrap and refrigerate for 1 to 2 hours. Cut each into 1-inch rollups.
Nutrition: Calories: 309, Fat: 8, Carbs: 4, Protein: 10

445. Nacho Bites

Preparation Time: 15 minutes
Cooking Time: 10 minutes
Servings: 4
Ingredients:
Cooking spray
¾ cup low-sodium black beans, drained and rinsed
½ teaspoon hot sauce
¼ teaspoon salt
20 corn tortilla chips
½ cup shredded non-dairy cheese

Directions:
Preheat the oven to 400°F. Coat 2 baking sheets with cooking spray. Mix and toss beans, hot sauce, and salt. Mash until coarse.
Place tortilla chips. Topped the chip with black bean mixture and 1 teaspoon of cheese. Bake until the cheese has melted.
Nutrition: Calories: 290, Fat: 1, Carbs: 3, Protein: 19

446. Snack Pizza with Mushrooms

Preparation Time: 10 minutes
Cooking Time: 10 minutes
Servings: 4
Ingredients:
Cooking spray
6 button mushrooms, chopped
4 whole-wheat English muffins
1 cup jarred tomato sauce
½ cup shredded non-dairy cheese
Directions:
Preheat the oven to 350°F. Coat with cooking spray. Split each of the English muffins and place crust-side down on the prepared baking sheet, leaving about 1 inch between them. Top each with 2 tablespoons of tomato sauce and spread the sauce to the bread. Top the tomato sauce with 3 tablespoons of mushrooms, then 1 tablespoon of cheese. Bake until cheese has melted and the bread is slightly toasted. Remove and let it cool for 10 minutes before serving.
Nutrition: Calories: 219, Fat: 12, Carbs: 2, Protein: 5

447. Crab Dip

Preparation Time: 10 minutes
Cooking Time: 1 hour
Servings: 2
Ingredients:
2 ounces crabmeat
1 tablespoon lime zest, grated
½ tablespoon lime juice
2 tablespoons mayonnaise
2 green onions, chopped
Cooking spray
Directions:
Grease your slow cooker with the cooking spray, and mix the crabmeat with the lime zest, juice, and the other ingredients inside.
Put the lid on, cook on Low for 1 hour, divide into bowls, and serve as a party dip.
Nutrition: Calories: 209, Fat: 2, Carbs: 7, Protein: 14

448. Lemony Shrimp Dip

Preparation Time: 10 minutes
Cooking Time: 2 hours
Servings: 2
Ingredients:
3 ounces non-dairy cheese, soft
1 pound shrimp, peeled, deveined, and chopped
½ tablespoon balsamic vinegar
2 tablespoons mayonnaise
½ tablespoon lemon juice
A pinch salt and black pepper
1 tablespoon parsley, chopped
Directions:
In your slow cooker, mix the non-dairy cheese with the shrimp and the other ingredients, whisk, put the lid on, and cook on Low for 2 hours.
Divide into bowls and serve as a dip.

449. Squash Salsa

Preparation Time: 10 minutes
Cooking Time: 3 hours
Servings: 2
Ingredients:
1 cup butternut squash, peeled and cubed
1 cup cherry tomatoes, cubed
1 cup avocado, peeled, pitted, and cubed
½ tablespoon balsamic vinegar
½ tablespoon lemon juice
1 tablespoon lemon zest, grated
¼ cup veggie stock
1 tablespoon chives, chopped
A pinch rosemary, dried
A pinch sage, dried
A pinch salt and black pepper
Directions:
In your slow cooker, mix the squash with the tomatoes, avocado and the other ingredients, toss, put the lid on, and cook on Low for 3 hours.
Divide into bowls and serve as a snack.
Nutrition: Calories: 3886, Fat: 6, Carbs: 4, Protein: 12

450. Flavory Beans Spread

Preparation Time: 10 minutes
Cooking Time: 6 hours
Servings: 2
Ingredients:
1 cup canned black beans, drained
2 tablespoons tahini paste
½ teaspoon balsamic vinegar

¼ cup veggie stock

½ tablespoon olive oil

Directions:

In your slow cooker, mix the beans with the tahini paste and the other ingredients, toss, put the lid on, and cook on Low for 6 hours.

Transfer to your food processor, blend well, divide into bowls, and serve.

Nutrition: Calories: 432, Fat: 12, Carbs: 6, Protein: 4

451.   Cucumber Sandwich Bites

Preparation Time: 5 minutes

Cooking Time: 0 minutes

Servings: 12

Ingredients:

1 cucumber, sliced

8 slices whole-wheat bread

2 tablespoons cream cheese, soft

1 tablespoon chives, chopped

¼ cup avocado, peeled, pitted, and mashed

1 teaspoon mustard

Salt and black pepper, to taste

Directions:

Spread the mashed avocado on each bread slice, also spread the rest of the ingredients except the cucumber slices.

Divide the cucumber slices into the bread slices, cut each slice in thirds, arrange on a platter, and serve as an appetizer.

Nutrition: Calories: 187 Fat: 12.4 g. Fiber: 2.1 g. Carbs: 4.5 g. Protein: 8.2 g.

452.   Cucumber Rolls

Preparation Time: 5 minutes

Cooking Time: 0 minutes

Servings: 6

Ingredients:

1 big cucumber, sliced lengthwise

1 tablespoon parsley, chopped

8 ounce canned tuna, drained and mashed

Salt and black pepper, to taste

1 tsp. lime juice

Directions:

Arrange cucumber slices on a working surface, divide the rest of the ingredients, and roll.

Arrange all the rolls on a platter and serve as an appetizer.

Nutrition: Calories: 200 Fat: 6 g. Fiber: 3.4 g. Carbs: 7.6 g. Protein: 3.5 g.

453.   Olives and Cheese Stuffed Tomatoes

Preparation Time: 10 minutes

Cooking Time: 0 minutes

Servings: 24

Ingredients:

24 cherry tomatoes, top cut off, and insides scooped out

2 tablespoons olive oil

¼ teaspoon red pepper flakes

½ cup feta cheese, crumbled

2 tablespoons black olive paste

¼ cup mint, torn

Directions:

In a bowl, mix the olives paste with the rest of the ingredients, except the cherry tomatoes, and whisk well. Stuff the cherry tomatoes with this mix, arrange them all on a platter, and serve as an appetizer.

Nutrition: Calories: 136 Fat: 8.6 g. Fiber: 4.8 g. Carbs: 5.6 g. Protein: 5.1 g.

454.   Tomato and Chives Salsa

Preparation Time: 5 minutes

Cooking Time: 0 minutes

Servings: 6

Ingredients:

1 garlic clove, minced

4 tablespoon olive oil

5 tomatoes, cubed

1 tablespoon balsamic vinegar

¼ cup basil, chopped

1 tablespoon parsley, chopped

1 tablespoon chives, chopped

Salt and black pepper, to taste

Pita chips, for serving

Directions:

In a bowl, mix the tomatoes with the garlic and the rest of the ingredients except the pita chips, stir, divide into small cups, and serve with the pita chips on the side.

Nutrition: Calories: 160 Fat: 13.7 g. Fiber: 5.5 g. Carbs: 10.1 g. Protein: 2.2 g.

455.   Chili Mango and Watermelon Salsa

Preparation Time: 5 minutes

Cooking Time: 0 minutes

Servings: 12

Ingredients:

1 red tomato, chopped

Salt and black pepper, to taste
1 cup watermelon, seedless, peeled and cubed
1 red onion, chopped
2 mangos, peeled and chopped
2 chili peppers, chopped
¼ cup cilantro, chopped
3 tablespoon lime juice
Pita chips, for serving

Directions:

In a bowl, mix the tomato with the watermelon, the onion, and the rest of the ingredients, except the pita chips, and toss well.

Divide the mix into small cups and serve with pita chips on the side.

Nutrition: Calories: 62 Fat: 4g. Fiber: 1.3 g. Carbs: 3.9 g. Protein: 2.3 g.

456. Creamy Spinach and Shallots Dip

Preparation Time: 10 minutes
Cooking Time: 0 minutes
Servings: 4
Ingredients:
1 pound spinach, roughly chopped
2 shallots, chopped
2 tablespoons mint, chopped
¾ cup nondairy cheese, soft
Salt and black pepper, to taste

Directions:

In a blender, combine the spinach with the shallots and the rest of the ingredients, then pulse well.

Divide into small bowls and serve as a party dip.

Nutrition: Calories: 204 Fat: 11.5 g. Fiber: 3.1 g. Carbs: 4.2 g. Protein: 5.9 g.

457. Maple   Lemon   Tempeh Cubes

Preparation Time:0
Cooking Time: 30 minutes
Servings: 2-3 servings
Ingredients:
Fresh ground black pepper
¼ teaspoon of powdered garlic
¼ teaspoon of dried basil
2 teaspoons of water
1-2 teaspoons of Bragg's Liquid Aminos or low-sodium tamari
2 teaspoons of maple syrup
3 Tablespoons of lemon juice
2-3 teaspoons of coconut oil

1 package of tempeh
Directions:

Heat your oven to 4000F. Then chop your tempeh into tiny squares. Put your coconut oil in a non-stick skillet and heat over medium-high heat. Once the oil becomes hot and melts. Add tempeh and let it cook for about 2-4 minutes on one of its sides or until you see that the tempeh color has turned to golden brown from the bottom. Turn the tempeh over and let it cook for additional 2-4 minutes.

When the tempeh is browning, you will have to mix the black pepper, garlic, basil, water, tamari, syrup, maple, and lemon juice. Then sauté it for 1-2 minutes. At this point, the tempeh should already be nice and brown on its 2 sides. Once sautéed, the tempeh can be served. However, if you want it to be a little crunchy, you can put it on a baking sheet and bake inside the oven for 15-20 minutes. Then, remove it from the oven and place in a plate to serve.

Nutrition: 308 Calories, 21g Protein, 22g Carbohydrate, 17 g Fat, Sugar: 5g , Fiber: 9g

458. Mini Mac in a Bowl

Preparation Time: 5 minutes
Cooking Time: 15 minutes
Servings: 1
Ingredients:
5 ounce of lean ground beef
Two tablespoons of diced white or yellow onion.
1/8 teaspoon of onion powder
1/8 teaspoon of white vinegar
1 ounce of dill pickle slices
One teaspoon sesame seed
3 cups of shredded Romaine lettuce
Cooking spray
Two tablespoons reduced-fat shredded cheddar cheese
Two tablespoons of Wish-bone light thousand island as dressing

Directions:

Place a lightly greased small skillet on fire to heat,
Add your onion to cook for about 2-3 minutes,
Next, add the beef and allow cooking until it's brown
Next, mix your vinegar and onion powder with the dressing,
Finally, top the lettuce with the cooked meat and sprinkle cheese on it, add your pickle slices.
Drizzle the mixture with the sauce and sprinkle the sesame seeds also.

Your mini mac in a bowl is ready for consumption.
Nutrition: Calories: 150Protein: 21 gCarbohydrates: 32 gFats: 19 g

459.   Cilantro   and Cranberry Quinoa Salad

Preparation Time: 10 minutes
Cooking Time: 20 minutes, Additional Time: 2 Hours
Servings: 6
Ingredients:
Ground pepper and salt to taste
½ cup of dried cranberries
½ cup of minced carrots
¼ cup of toasted sliced almonds
1 lime, to be juiced
¼ cup of chopped fresh cilantro
1 ½ teaspoon of curry powder
1 small red onion, should be finely chopped
¼ cup of yellow bell pepper, to be chopped
¼ cup of red bell pepper, to be chopped
1 cup of uncooked quinoa, should be rinsed
1 ½ cups of water
Directions:

Get a saucepan and pour the water inside and get a lid to cover it. Place it over high heat and let it boil after which you should pour the quinoa, reduce the heat to low, and let it simmer until the water evaporates in about 15-20 minutes. Whisk it into a mixing bowl and place in the refrigerator to get cold. As soon as it becomes cold, stir in the cranberries, carrots, sliced almond, lime juice, cilantro, curry powder, red onion, yellow bell pepper, red bell pepper. Then season to taste with pepper and salt. Let it chill before you serve.
Nutrition: 176.2 Calories, 5.4g Protein, 31.6g Carbohydrate, 3.9 g Fat, Sodium: 92.6mg , Cholesterol: 0mg , Sugars: 13.1g

460.   Mediterranean   Bean Salad

Preparation Time: 2 hours and 20 minutes
CookingTime: 0
Servings: 4
Ingredients:
½ teaspoon of salt or as desired to taste
3 tablespoons of extra virgin olive oil
1 teaspoon of capers, should be rinsed and drained
½ cup of chopped fresh parsley
¼ cup of chopped red onion

1 medium-size tomato, to be chopped
1 lemon, should be zested and juiced
1 (15 ounce) can of kidney beans, should be drained
1 (15.5 ounce) can of garbanzo beans, should be drained
Directions:
Get a large bowl and mix together the salt, olive oil, capers, parsley, onion, tomato, lemon juice, kidney beans, and garbanzo beans. Cover with a lid and place in the refrigerator for about 2 hours. Stir very well before you serve.
Nutrition: 328.9 Calories, 12.1g Protein, 46.6g Carbohydrate, 12 g Fat, Sodium: 874.1mg , Cholesterol: 0mg , Sugars: 1.3g

461.   Megan's Granola

Preparation Time: 20 minutes
Cooking Time: 20 minutes
Servings: 30
Total Time: 40 minutes
Ingredients:
2 cups of sweetened dried cranberries or raisins
1 tablespoon of vanilla extract
1 tablespoon of ground cinnamon
1 cup of vegetable oil
¾ cup of honey
¼ cup of maple syrup
½ cup of brown sugar
1 ½ teaspoon of salt
1 cup of finely chopped walnuts
1 cup of finely chopped pecans
1 cup of finely chopped almonds
1 cup sunflower seeds
1 ½ cups of oat bran
1 ½ cups of wheat germ
 8 cups rolled oats
Directions:
Let your oven preheat to 3250F (1650C). Get 2 baking sheets and line with aluminum foil or parchment
Get a large bowl and combine the walnuts, pecans, almonds, sunflower seeds, oat bran, wheat germ, and oats inside. Next is to get a saucepan and stir together the vanilla, cinnamon, oil, honey, maple syrup, brown sugar, and salt. Place over medium heat and let it boil, then pour on top of the dry ingredients and stir to have a coat. Let the mixture spread in an even manner on top of the baking sheets.
Next is to bake in the already preheated oven until it becomes toasted and crispy in about 20 minutes.

Only stir once when half done. Once toasted, let it cool and stir in the cranberries or raisins before you store in the airtight container.

Nutrition: 368.6 Calories, 8.3g Protein, 45g Carbohydrate, 20 g Fat, Sodium: 121.9mg , Cholesterol: 0mg , Sugars: 19.5g

462. Egg Stir Fry and Tomato

Preparation Time: 10 minutes
Cooking Time: 5 minutes
Servings: 3
Ingredients:
2 medium (4 – 1/8" long) green onions, should be thinly sliced
4 eaches of ripe tomatoes, should be sliced into wedges
6 large eggs, should be beaten
2 tablespoons of avocado oil or more if desired
Directions:
Put 1 tablespoon of avocado oil in a skillet or wok and heat over medium heat. Cook and stir the eggs while in the eggs to thoroughly cook through in just a minute. Then, transfer the eggs inside a clean plate. You should pour the 1 teaspoon left of the avocado oil inside the wok, cook, and continue to stir the tomatoes for 2 minutes or until its liquid evaporates. Place the eggs back inside the wok and add green onions; you should continue to stir while cooking until the eggs are thoroughly cooked, which should take about 30 seconds.

Nutrition: 264.2 Calories, 14.5g Protein, 9.2g Carbohydrate, 19.7 g Fat, Sodium: 151.5mg , Cholesterol: 372mg , Sugars: 6.2g

463. Homemade Peanut Butter

Preparation Time: 5 minutes
Cookimg Time: 0
Servings: 25
Ingredients:
2 pounds of honey roasted peanuts
2 tablespoons of peanut oil
Directions:
Get a food processor and pour the peanut oil inside its bowl. Switch ON the processor. As its blade spins, add the peanuts in a gradual process. Let the food processor work on the peanuts until they become smooth in about 2 minutes. Scrape the sides of the bowl that might have the smooth peanut extracts.

Put in an airtight container and store inside the refrigerator.

Nutrition: 190.6 Calories, 12.7g Protein, 12.7g Carbohydrate, 10.1 g Fat, Sodium: 181mg , Cholesterol: 0mg , Sugars: 5.4g

464. Mini Frittatas with Quinoa

Preparation Time: 20 minutes
Cooking Time: 45 minutes, Additional Time: 5 minutes
Servings: 6
Ingredients:
¼ teaspoon of ground white pepper
2 tablespoons of grated Parmesan cheese
¼ cup of chopped fresh parsley
½ cup of diced ham
1 cup of shredded Swiss cheese
1 cup of shredded zucchini
2 large egg whites
2 large eggs
¾ cup of quinoa, should be rinsed and drained
1 ½ cups of water
Directions:
Preheat your oven to 4000F (2000C). Get 6 muffin cups and grease.
Get a saucepan and add water and quinoa, then let it boil. Reduce the heat to medium-low, cover with a lid, simmer until it is absorbed, and the quinoa becomes tender in about 15-20 minutes.
Get a large bowl and combine white pepper, Parmesan cheese, parsley, ham, Swiss cheese, zucchini, egg whites, eggs, and cooked quinoa, make sure to mix very well to have an even combination. Transfer the mixture on top of all the prepared muffin cups
Finally, bake in the preheated oven until the frittata's edges become golden brown in approximately 30 minutes. Let it cool for about 5 minutes before you serve. You can either serve hot or cold.

Nutrition: 213.3 Calories, 14g Protein, 15.5g Carbohydrate, 10.5 g Fat, Sodium: 256mg , Cholesterol: 86.3mg , Sugars: 0.8g

465. Tomatillo and Green Chili Pork Stew

Preparation Time: 10 minutes
Cooking Time: 20 minutes
Servings: 4
Ingredients:

2 scallions, chopped
2 cloves of garlic
1 lb. tomatillos, trimmed and chopped
8 large romaine or green lettuce leaves, divided
2 serrano chilies, seeds, and membranes
½ tsp of dried Mexican oregano (or you can use regular oregano)
1 ½ lb. of boneless pork loin, to be cut into bite-sized cubes
¼ cup of cilantro, chopped
¼ tablespoon (each) salt and paper
1 jalapeno, seeds and membranes to be removed and thinly sliced
1 cup of sliced radishes
4 lime wedges

Directions:

Combine scallions, garlic, tomatillos, 4 lettuce leaves, serrano chilies, and oregano in a blender. Then puree until smooth

Put pork and tomatillo mixture in a medium pot. 1-inch of puree should cover the pork; if not, add water until it covers it. Season with pepper & salt, and cover it simmers. Simmer on heat for approximately 20 minutes.

Now, finely shred the remaining lettuce leaves.

When the stew is done cooking, garnish with cilantro, radishes, finely shredded lettuce, sliced jalapenos, and lime wedges.

Nutrition: Calories: 370 Protein: 36g Carbohydrate: 14g Fat: 19 g

466. Optavia Cloud Bread

Preparation Time: 25 minutes
Cooking Time: 35 minutes
Servings: 3
Ingredients:

½ cup of Fat-free 0% Plain Greek Yogurt (4.4 0z)
3 Eggs, Separated
16 teaspoon Cream of Tartar
1 Packet sweetener (a granulated sweetener just like stevia)

Directions:

For about 30 minutes before making this meal, place the Kitchen Aid Bowl and the whisk attachment in the freezer.

Preheat your oven to 30 degrees

Remove the mixing bowl and whisk attachment from the freezer

Separate the eggs. Now put the egg whites in the Kitchen Aid Bowl, and they should be in a different medium-sized bowl.

In the medium-sized bowl containing the yolks, mix in the sweetener and yogurt.

In the bowl containing the egg white, add in the cream of tartar. Beat this mixture until the egg whites turn to stiff peaks.

Now, take the egg yolk mixture and carefully fold it into the egg whites. Be cautious and avoid over-stirring.

Place baking paper on a baking tray and spray with cooking spray.

Scoop out 6 equally-sized "blobs" of the "dough" onto the parchment paper.

Bake for about 25-35 minutes (make sure you check when it is 25 minutes, in some ovens, they are done at this timestamp). You will know they are done as they will get brownish at the top and have some crack.

Most people like them cold against being warm

Most people like to re-heat in a toast oven or toaster to get them a little bit crispy.

Your serving size should be about 2 pieces.

Nutrition: Calories: 234 Protein: 23g Carbs: 5g Fiber: 8g Sodium: 223g

Chapter 10:

After- Dinner Snacks

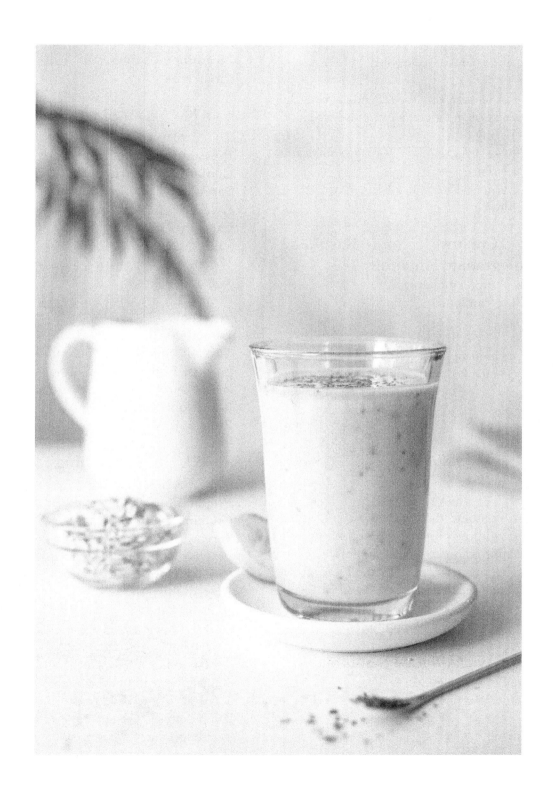

467. Vegan Feta Artichoke Dip

Preparation Time: 10 minutes
Cooking Time: 30 minutes
Servings: 8
Ingredients:
8 ounces artichoke hearts, drained and quartered
¾ cup basil, chopped
¾ cup green olives, pitted and chopped
1 cup nondairy cheese, grated
5 ounce Vegan feta cheese, crumbled
Directions:
In your food processor, mix the artichokes with the basil and the rest of the ingredients, pulse well, and transfer to a baking dish.
Put into the oven, bake at 375°F for 30 minutes and serve as a party dip.
Nutrition: Calories: 186; Fat: 12.4 g; Fiber: 0.9 g; Carbs: 2.6 g; Protein: 1.5 g

468. Creamy Raspberry Pomegranate Smoothie

Preparation Time: 5 minutes
Cooking Time: 5 minutes
Serving: 1
Ingredients:
1 ½ cups pomegranate juice
½ cup unsweetened coconut milk
1 scoop vanilla protein powder (plant-based if you need it to be dairy-free)
2 packed cups fresh baby spinach
1 cup frozen raspberries
1 frozen banana (see Tip)
1 to 2 tablespoons freshly compressed lemon juice
Directions:
In a blender, combine the pomegranate juice and coconut milk. Add the protein powder and spinach. Give these a whirl to break down the spinach.
Add the raspberries, banana, and lemon juice, then top it off with ice. Blend until smooth and frothy.
Nutrition: Calories: 303 Total fat: 3g Cholesterol: 0mg Fiber: 2g Protein: 15g Sodium: 165mg

469. Avocado Kale Smoothie

Preparation Time: 5 minutes
Cooking Time: 0 minutes
Servings: 3
Level of Difficulty: Easy
Category: Green/Healthy Fat:
Ingredients:
1 cup water

½ Seville orange, peeled
1 avocado
1 cucumber, peeled
1 cup kale
1 cup ice cubes
Directions:
Toss all your ingredients into your blender, then process till smooth and creamy. Serve immediately and enjoy.
Nutrition: Calories: 160 Fat: 13.3g Carbs: 11.6g Protein: 2.4g

470. Apple Kale Cucumber Smoothie

Preparation Time: 5 minutes
Cooking Time: 0 minutes
Servings: 1
Level of Difficulty: Easy
Category: Green
Ingredients:
¾ cup water
½ green apple, diced
¾ cup kale
½ cucumber
Directions:
Toss all your ingredients into your blender, then process till smooth and creamy. Serve immediately and enjoy.
Nutrition: Calories: 86 Fat: 0.5g Carbs: 21.7g Protein: 1.9g

471. Refreshing Cucumber Smoothie

Preparation Time: 5 minutes
Cooking Time: 0 minutes
Servings: 2
Level of Difficulty: Easy
Category: Green
Ingredients:
1 cup ice cubes
20 drops liquid stevia
2 fresh lime, peeled and halved
1 teaspoon lime zest, grated
1 cucumber, chopped
1 avocado, pitted and peeled
2 cups kale
1 tablespoon creamed coconut
¾ cup coconut water

Directions:

Toss all your ingredients into your blender, then process till smooth and creamy. Serve immediately and enjoy.

Nutrition: Calories: 313 Fat: 25.1g Carbs: 24.7g Protein: 4.9g

472. Cauliflower Veggie Smoothie

Preparation Time: 5 minutes
Cooking Time: 5 minutes
Servings: 4
Level of Difficulty: Easy
Category: Green
Ingredients:
1 zucchini, peeled and chopped
1 Seville orange, peeled
1 apple, diced
1 banana
1 cup kale
½ cup cauliflower
Directions:
Toss all your ingredients into your blender, then process till smooth and creamy. Serve immediately and enjoy.
Nutrition: Calories: 71 Fat: 0.3g Carbs: 18.3g Protein: 1.3g

473. Soursop Smoothie

Preparation Time: 5 minutes
Cooking Time: 0 minutes
Servings: 2
Level of Difficulty: Easy
Category: Green
Ingredients:
3 quartered frozen Burro Bananas
1 ½ cups Homemade Coconut Milk
¼ cup Walnuts
1 teaspoon Sea Moss Gel
1 teaspoon ground Ginger
1 teaspoon Soursop Leaf Powder
1 handful of kale
Directions:
Prepare and put all ingredients in a blender or a food processor. Blend it well until you reach a smooth consistency. Serve and enjoy your Soursop Smoothie!
Nutrition: Calories: 213 Fat: 3.1g Carbs: 6g Protein: 8g

474. Coconut Smoothie

Preparation Time: 5 minutes
Cooking Time: 0 minutes
Servings: 1
Level of Difficulty: Easy
Category: Healthy Fat:
Ingredients:
1 sachet Lean and Green Essential Creamy Vanilla Shake
6 ounces unsweetened almond milk
6 ounces diet ginger ale
2 tablespoons unsweetened coconut, shredded
¼ teaspoon rum extract
½ cup ice
Directions:
In a small blender, place all ingredients and pulse until smooth. Transfer the smoothie into a serving glass and serve immediately.
Nutrition: Calories: 120 Fat: 6.2g Carbohydrates: 15.9g Protein: 15g

475. Black Bean Burgers

Preparation Time: 15 minutes
Cooking Time: 10 minutes
Servings: 8 burgers
Level of Difficulty: Normal
Category: Green
Ingredients:
½ cup dried breadcrumbs
½ cup sun-dried tomatoes in oil
2 tablespoons olive oil
½ medium red onion
1 tablespoon paprika
1 ½ tablespoon cumin
½ tablespoon salt
1 can black beans
1 egg
½ cup rolled oats
Directions:
Wash and drain the black beans. Blend with a hand blender and place it in a big mixing bowl. Conversely, crush the beans with a fork/masher.
Dice the red onion and sundried tomatoes, and add them to the dish. Then, add some salt, chickens, cumin, oats, paprika, olive oil, etc. Give a nice stir to it.
Finally, put some of the breadcrumbs until you're left with a good, firm mixture. If you don't need to use all the breadcrumbs, that's cool. Sculpt the paste into

patties for burgers. If it is too sticky, wet your hands a little.

Fry in a pan with a little oil, or place on a grill. Cook on both sides within 5 minutes, turning occasionally. Serve whatever you fancy with your favorite burger

Ingredients: a bun, lettuce, tomato, cheese!

Nutrition: Calories: 95 Carbs: 18g Fat: 1g Protein: 6g

476.   Lean and Green Smoothie

Preparation Time: 5 minutes

Cooking Time: 0 minutes

Servings: 1

Ingredients:

2 ½ cups kale leaves

¾ cup chilled apple juice

1 cup cubed pineapple

½ cup frozen green grapes

½ cup chopped apple

Directions:

Place the pineapple, apple juice, apple, frozen seedless grapes, and kale leaves in a blender.

Cover and blend until it's smooth.

Smoothie is ready and can be garnished with halved grapes if you wish.

Nutrition: Calories: 81 Protein: 2 g Carbohydrates: 19 g Fat: 1 g

477.   Strawberry   Cheesecake Minis

Preparation Time: 30 minutes.

Cooking Time: 120 minutes.

Servings: 5.

Ingredients:

1 cup coconut oil.

1 cup coconut butter.

½ cup strawberries, sliced.

½ teaspoon lime juice.

2 tablespoons vegan cream cheese, full fat.

Stevia, to taste.

Directions:

Blend your strawberries together.

Soften your vegan cream cheese, and then add in your coconut butter.

Combine all ingredients together, and then pour your mixture into silicone molds.

Freeze for at least 2 hours before serving.

Nutrition: Calories: 372. Protein: 1 g. Fat: 41 g. Carbohydrates: 2 g.

478.   Cocoa Brownies

Preparation Time: 10 minutes.

Cooking Time: 30 minutes.

Servings: 12.

Ingredients:

1 egg.

2 tablespoons vegan butter, grass-fed.

2 teaspoons vanilla extract, pure.

¼ teaspoon baking powder.

¼ cup cocoa powder.

1/3 cup heavy cream.

¾ cup almond butter.

Pinch sea salt.

Directions:

Break your egg into a bowl, whisking until smooth.

Add in all of your wet ingredients, mixing well.

Mix all dry ingredients into a bowl.

Sift your dry ingredients into your wet ingredients, mixing to form a batter.

Use a baking pan, greasing it before pouring in your mixture.

Heat your oven to 350°F and bake for 25 minutes.

Allow it to cool before slicing and serve at room temperature or warm.

Nutrition: Calories: 184. Protein: 1 g. Fat: 20 g. Carbohydrates: 1 g.

479.   Chocolate Orange Bites

Preparation Time: 20 minutes.

Cooking Time: 120 minutes.

Servings: 10.

Ingredients:

ounces coconut oil.

4 tablespoons cocoa powder.

¼ teaspoon orange extract.

Stevia, to taste.

Directions:

Melt half of your coconut oil using a double boiler, and then add in your stevia and orange extract.

Use candy molds, pouring the mixture into it. Fill each mold halfway, and then place in the fridge until they set.

Melt the other half of your coconut oil, stirring in your cocoa powder and stevia, making sure that the mixture is smooth with no lumps.

Pour into your molds, filling them up all the way, and then allow it to set in the fridge before serving.

Nutrition: Calories: 188. Protein: 1 g. Fat: 21 g. Carbohydrates: 5 g.

480.   Black Bean Tacos

Preparation Time: 15 minutes
Cooking Time: 10 minutes
Servings: 4
Ingredients:
1 cup of shredded lettuce
1 avocado, should be sliced
1 tomato, should be diced
2 ounces of shredded Mexican cheese, blend
6 eaches of taco shells
½ teaspoon of ground cumin
½ teaspoon of chili powder
½ teaspoon of garlic powder
1 (7 ounces) can of green salsa (salsa verde)
1 (15 ounce) can of black beans, should be rinsed and drained
1 small onion, should be chopped
1 tablespoon of olive oil
Directions:
Get a saucepan and pour in the olive oil, which should be heated over medium-low heat. Then, cook onion in the hot oil until it becomes tender in about 5 minutes. Stir cumin, chili powder, garlic powder, green salsa, black beans with the onion. Lower the heat to low and cook the mixture till it becomes thicken in about 5-10 minutes.
Serve with shredded lettuce, avocado, tomato, Mexican cheese blend, and taco shells.
Nutrition: 402.1 Calories, 13g Protein, 43.9g Carbohydrate, 20.5 g Fat, Sodium: 778.1mg , Cholesterol: 13.5mg , Sugars: 4.4g

481.   Sabich Sandwich

Preparation Time: 5 minutes
Cooking Time: 15 minutes
Serving: 2
Ingredients:
2 tomatoes
Olive oil
½ lb. eggplant
¼ cucumber
1 tablespoon lemon
1 tablespoon parsley
¼ head cabbage
2 tablespoons wine vinegar
2 pita bread
½ cup hummus
¼ tahini sauce
2 hard-boiled eggs

Directions:
In a skillet fry eggplant slices until tender
In a bowl add tomatoes, cucumber, parsley, lemon juice and season salad
In another bowl toss cabbage with vinegar
In each pita pocket add hummus, eggplant and drizzle tahini sauce
Top with eggs, tahini sauce
Nutrition: Calories: 269   Total Carbohydrate: 2 g Cholesterol: 3 mg Total Fat: 14 g Fiber: 2 g Protein: 7 g Sodium: 183 mg

Chapter 11:

Fueling Hacks Recipes

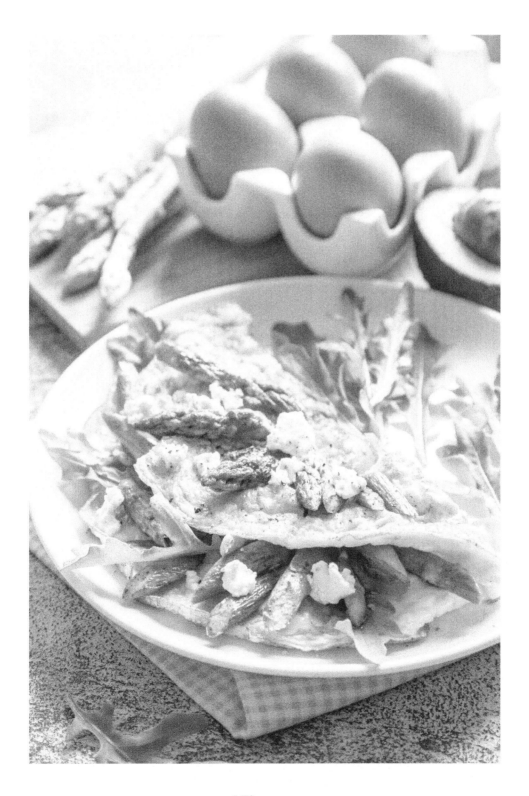

482. Asparagus Green Scramble

Preparation Time: 5 minutes
Cooking Time: 6 minutes
Servings: 2
Ingredients:
3 eggs
1 Portobello mushroom, chopped
2 garlic cloves, chopped
1/2 cup spinach
4 asparagus, trimmed, diced
Sea salt to taste
Cayenne pepper to taste
1 tbsp olive oil
Directions:
In a bowl, whisk the eggs with salt and cayenne pepper.
In a skillet, add the oil and pour in the egg mix.
Cook for 1 minute.
Add the spinach, mushroom, asparagus, and garlic.
Stir for 4 minutes. Serve.
Nutrition: Carbohydrates: 3 g, Fat: 6 g, Protein: 13 g

483. No Bake Optavia Fueling Peanut Butter Brownies

Preparation Time: 5 minutes
Cooking Time: 30 minutes
Servings: 6
Ingredients:
3 tablespoons peanut butter
1 cup water
6 packets Optavia Double Chocolate Brownie Fueling
Directions:
Put all ingredients in a bowl and mix until all elements are well incorporated.
Pour into silicone molds and place in the freezer.
Freeze for 30 minutes before eating.
Nutrition: Calories per serving: 906 Cal, Protein: 8.7 g, Carbohydrates: 157 g, Fat: 31.8 g, Sugar: 1.5 g

484. Peanut Butter Brownie Ice Cream Sandwiches

Preparation Time: 2 minutes
Cooking Time: 2 minutes
Servings: 2
Ingredients:
1 packet Medifast Brownie Mix
3 tablespoons water
1 Peanut Butter Crunch Bar or any bar of your choice
2 tablespoons Peanut Butter Powder
1 tablespoon water
2 tablespoons cool whip
Directions:
Melt the Brownie Mix with water.
Add in the Peanut Butter Crunch until a dough is formed.
Spoon 4 dough balls on a plate and flatten using the palm of your hands.
Make sure that the dough is 1/4 inch thick.
Place in a microwave oven and cook for 2 minutes.
Meanwhile, mix the Peanut Butter Powder and water to form a paste. Add cool whip. Set aside in the fridge to chill for at least 1 hour.
Take the cookies out from the microwave oven and allow to cool.
Once cooled, spoon the Peanut Butter ice cream in between two cookies.
Serve immediately.
Nutrition: Calories per serving: 410 Cal, Protein: 8.3 g, Carbohydrates: 57.6 g, Fat: 13.2 g, Sugar: 5.3g

485. Cranberry Salad

Preparation Time: 5 minutes
Cooking Time: 5 minutes
Servings: 2
Ingredients:
1 Sugar free cranberry jello pack (1/2 cup for snacks allowed)
1/2 cup celery chopped (1 green)
7 Half Cut Walnut (1 snack)
Directions:
Jello mix according to the instructions of the box.
Attach walnuts and celery.
Allow setting.
Shake until serving.
Requires servings in 4-1/2 cups.
Nutrition: Fats: 11 g, Sodium: 73 mg, Potassium: 212 mg, Carbohydrates: 54 g, Protein: 4.1 g

486. Chicken Salad With Pineapple And Pecans

Preparation Time: 10 minutes
Cooking Time: 5 minutes
Servings: 4
Ingredients:
(6-ounce) Boneless, skinless, cooked and cubed chicken breast
Tablespoons of celery hacked
Cut 1/4 cup of pineapple

1/4 cup orange peeled segments
Tablespoon of pecans hacked
1/4 cup seedless grapes
Salt and black chili pepper, to taste
Cups cut from roman lettuce

Directions:

Put chicken, celery, pineapple, grapes, pecans, and raisins in a medium dish.

Kindly blend until mixed with a spoon, then season with salt and pepper.

Create a bed of lettuce on a plate.

Cover with mixture of chicken and serve.

Nutrition: Calories: 386 Cal, Carbohydrates: 20 g, Fat: 19 g , Protein: 25 g

487.   Zucchini Fritters

Preparation Time: 15 minutes
Cooking Time: 10 minutes
Servings: 4
Ingredients:

1 1/2 pound of grated zucchini
1 Tsp. of salt
1/4 cup of grated Parmesan
1/4 cup of flour
2 cloves of minced garlic
2 Tbsp of olive oil
1 large egg
Freshly ground black pepper and kosher salt to taste

Directions:

Put the grated zucchini into a colander over the sink Add your salt and toss it to mix properly, then leave it to settle for about 10 minutes.

Next, use a clean cheese cloth to drain the zucchini completely.

Combine drained zucchini, Parmesan, garlic, flour, and the beaten egg in a large bowl, mix, and season with pepper and salt.

Next, heat the olive oil in a skillet applying medium-high heat.

Use a tablespoon to scoop batter for each cake, put in the oil, and flatten using a spatula.

Allow to cook until the underside is richly golden brown, then flip over to the other side and cook.

Your delicious Zucchini fritters are ready to be served.

Nutrition: Total Fat: 12.0 g, Cholesterol: 101.9 mg, Sodium: 728.9 mg, Total Carbohydrate: 11.9 g, Dietary Fiber: 1.9 g, Sugars: 4.6 g, Protein: 8.6 g

488.   Healthy Broccoli Salad

Preparation Time: 5 minutes
Cooking Time: 25 minutes
Servings: 6
Ingredients:

3 cups broccoli, chopped
1 tbsp apple cider vinegar
1/2 cup Greek yogurt
2 tbsp sunflower seeds
3 bacon slices, cooked and chopped
1/3 cup onion, sliced
1/4 tsp. stevia

Directions:

In a mixing bowl, mix broccoli, onion, and bacon.

In a small bowl, mix yogurt, vinegar, and stevia and pour over broccoli mixture.

Stir to combine.

Sprinkle sunflower seeds on top of the salad.

Store salad in the refrigerator for 30 minutes.

Serve and enjoy.

Nutrition: Calories: 90 Cal,   Fat: 4.9   g, Carbohydrates: 5.4 g , Sugar: 2.5 g, Protein: 6.2 g, Cholesterol: 12 mg

489.   Optavia Biscuit Pizza

Preparation Time: 5 minutes
Cooking Time: 15 minutes
Servings: 2
Ingredients:

1 sachet Optavia Buttermilk Cheddar and Herb Biscuit
2 tablespoons water
1 tablespoon tomato sauce
1 tablespoon low fat cheese, shredded

Directions:

Preheat the oven or toaster to 3500F for 5 minutes.

In a bowl, stir the Optavia Buttermilk Cheddar and Herb Biscuit with water to form a thick paste. Spread into a thin circle on a baking tray lined with parchment paper.

Cook for 10 minutes to harden.

Once harden, spread tomato sauce on top and cheese.

Bake for another 5 minutes.

Nutrition: Calories per serving: 437 Cal, Protein: 9.5 g, Carbohydrates: 68.5 g, Fat: 5.3 g, Sugar: 4.3 g

490.   Greek Yogurt Cookie Dough

Preparation Time: 5 minutes
Cooking Time: 0
Servings: 1
Ingredients:
1, 53 oz. container of low-fat plain Greek yogurt
1 sachet of Optavia Essential Chewy Chocolate Chip Cookie
Directions:
Combine the Greek yogurt with the Chewy Chocolate Chip's contents and chill till the time of serving.
Per Serving: ½ Leaner , 1 Fueling

491.   Taco Salad

Preparation Time: 5 minutes
Cooking Time: 0
Servings: 1
Ingredients:
2 tablespoons of lime vinaigrette
2 tablespoons of Pico de Gallo
¼ cup of reduced-fat, shredded Mexican-blend cheese
½ medium orange bell pepper, should be chopped
5 oz. of extra-lean ground turkey, should be seasoned with ½ teaspoon of taco seasoning
2 cups of romaine lettuce
1 sachet of Optavia Puffed Ranch Snacks
Directions:
Get a medium-sized bowl, and combine pico de gallo, cheese, pepper, ground turkey, and lettuce together. Top salad with the dressing and Puffed Ranch Snacks and serve instantly.
Per Serving: 1 Healthy Fat , 3 Green , 1 Leaner

492.   Cheddar & Chive Savory Smashed Potato Waffles

Preparation Time: 5 minutes
Cooking Time: 10 minutes
Servings: 4
Ingredients:
Cooking Spray
¼ cup of chopped scallions
2 slices of turkey bacon, you will need to cook it with directions on the package before chopping into pieces
½ cup of liquid egg substitute
½ cup of shredded, reduced-fat cheddar cheese
½ cup of unsweetened cashew milk or almond

4 Sachets of Optavia Essential Roasted Garlic Creamy Smashed Potatoes
Optional Topping
¼ cup of low-fat, plain Greek yogurt (1 tablespoon per serving)
Directions:
Get a medium-size bowl to mix the egg substitute, cheese, milk, and Creamy Smashed Potatoes until they are all thoroughly combined. Then carefully fold the remnants of the ingredients.
Next is to pour the mixture inside a hot and lightly greased waffle iron, cover it with its lid and let it bake for 5-7 minutes when it should turn golden brown. Finally, remove the waffle from the waffle iron before serving.
Per Serving: 1 Condiment , 1 Fueling , ½ Lean

493.   Tiramisu Milkshake

Preparation Time: 5 minutes
Cooking Time: 10 minutes
Servings: 1
Ingredients:
2 tablespoons of pressurized whipped topping
2 tablespoons of sugar-free chocolate syrup
½ cup of unsweetened cashew milk or almond
6 oz. of plain low-fat Greek yogurt
½ cup of ice
1 sachet of Optavia Frosty Coffee Soft Serve Treat
Directions:
Get a blender and combine all of the ingredients inside, then blend until they become smooth.
Transfer the smooth mixture inside a mason jar or glass. Finally, dress with syrup before you top with whipped topping.
Per Serving: 2 ½ Condiments , 1 Fueling , ½ Leaner

494.   Yogurt Berry Bagels with Cream Cheese

Preparation Time: 20 minutes
Cooking Time: 0 minutes
Servings: 2
Ingredients:
1 oz. of light cream cheese
Cooking Spray
½ teaspoon of baking powder
2 tablespoon of liquid egg substitute
1/3 cup of unsweetened, cashew milk or original almond
2 sachets of Optavia Essential Yogurt Berry Blast Smoothie

Directions:

Preheat your oven to 3500F.

Get a medium-sized bowl to combine baking powder, egg substitute, milk, and packets of Yogurt Berry Blast Smoothie.

Get 4 lightly-greased slots of donut pans to divide the mixture gotten.

Bake till the mixture is set in about 12-15 minutes.

Let it cool a little before you serve. Serve with cream cheese.

Per Serving: 1 ½ Condiment , 1 Fueling , ½ Healthy Fat

495.   Chicken Caesar Salad

Preparation Time: 20 minutes

Cooking Time: 0 minutes

Servings: 1

Ingredients:

2 tablespoons of light Caesar dressing

2 tablespoons of shredded parmesan cheese

½ cup of grape or cherry tomatoes, should be halved

6 oz. of cooked chicken breast, sliced or cubed

2 cups of romaine lettuce

1 sachet of Optavia Puffed Ranch Snacks

Directions:

Get a medium-size bowl to combine cheese, tomatoes, chicken breast, and lettuce.

Top the salad with Puffed Ranch Snacks and dressing and serve instantly.

Per Serving: 2 Condiments , 3 Green , 1 Healthy Fat , 1 Leaner , 1 Optional Snack

496.   Sriracha Butter Popcorn

Preparation Time: 10 minutes

Cooking Time: 0 minutes

Servings: 1

Ingredients:

Pinch of stevia

1 teaspoon sriracha

1 teaspoon of unsalted butter, should be melted

1 sachet of Optavia Sharp Cheddar & Sour Cream Popcorn

Directions:

Mix stevia, sriracha, and butter.

Get a quart-size mall bowl or resealable plastic bag and put the Sharp Cheddar & Sour Cream Popcorn. Then, trickle with butter mixture.

Mix gently or toss to get evenly coat popcorn

Per Serving: 1 Condiment , 1 Optional Snack , 2/3 Healthy Fat

497.   Chocolate Bars

Preparation Time: 10 minutes

Cooking Time: 20 minutes

Servings: 16

Ingredients:

15 oz cream cheese, softened

15 oz unsweetened dark chocolate

1 tsp vanilla

10 drops liquid stevia

Directions:

Grease 8-inch square dish and set aside.

In a saucepan dissolve chocolate over low heat.

Add stevia and vanilla and stir well.

Remove pan from heat and set aside.

Add cream cheese into the blender and blend until smooth.

Add melted chocolate mixture into the cream cheese and blend until just combined.

Transfer mixture into the prepared dish and spread evenly and place in the refrigerator until firm.

Slice and serve.

Nutrition: Calories: 230 Fat: 24 g Carbs: 7.5 g Sugar: 0.1 g Protein: 6 g Cholesterol: 29 mg

498.   Blueberry Muffins

Preparation Time: 15 minutes

Cooking Time: 35 minutes

Servings: 12

Ingredients:

2 eggs

1/2 cup fresh blueberries

1 cup heavy cream

2 cups almond flour

1/4 tsp lemon zest

1/2 tsp lemon extract

1 tsp baking powder

5 drops stevia

1/4 cup butter, melted

Directions:

heat the cooker to 350 F. Line muffin tin with cupcake liners and set aside.

Add eggs into the bowl and whisk until mix.

Add remaining ingredients and mix to combine.

Pour mixture into the prepared muffin tin and bake for 25 minutes.

Serve and enjoy.

Nutrition: Calories: 190 Fat: 17 g Carbs: 5 g Sugar: 1 g Protein: 5 g Cholesterol: 55 mg

499. Chia Pudding

Preparation Time: 20 minutes
Cooking Time: 0 minutes
Servings: 2
Ingredients:
4 tbsp chia seeds
1 cup unsweetened coconut milk
1/2 cup raspberries
Directions:
Add raspberry and coconut milk into a blender and blend until smooth.
Pour mixture into the glass jar.
Add chia seeds in a jar and stir well.
Seal the jar with a lid and shake well and place in the refrigerator for 3 hours.
Serve chilled and enjoy.
Nutrition: Calories: 360 Fat: 33 g Carbs: 13 g Sugar: 5 g Protein: 6 g Cholesterol: 0 mg

500. Avocado Pudding

Preparation Time: 20 minutes
Cooking Time: 0 minutes
Servings: 8
Ingredients:
2 ripe avocados, pitted and cut into pieces
1 tbsp fresh lime juice
14 oz can coconut milk
2 tsp liquid stevia
2 tsp vanilla
Directions:
Inside the blender Add all ingredients and blend until smooth.
Serve immediately and enjoy.
Nutrition: Calories: 317 Fat: 30 g Carbs: 9 g Sugar: 0.5 g Protein: 3 g Cholesterol: 0 mg

501. Delicious Brownie Bites

Preparation Time: 20 minutes
Cooking Time: 0 minutes
Servings: 13
Ingredients:
1/4 cup unsweetened chocolate chips
1/4 cup unsweetened cocoa powder
1 cup pecans, chopped
1/2 cup almond butter
1/2 tsp vanilla
1/4 cup monk fruit sweetener
1/8 tsp pink salt

Directions:
Add pecans, sweetener, vanilla, almond butter, cocoa powder, and salt into the food processor and process until well combined.
Transfer brownie mixture into the large bowl. Add chocolate chips and fold well.
Make small round shape balls from brownie mixture and place onto a baking tray.
Place in the freezer for 20 minutes.
Serve and enjoy.
Nutrition: Calories: 108 Fat: 9 g Carbs: 4 g Sugar: 1 g Protein: 2 g Cholesterol: 0 mg

502. Pumpkin Balls

Preparation Time: 15 minutes
Cooking Time: 0 minutes
Servings: 18
Ingredients:
1 cup almond butter
5 drops liquid stevia
2 tbsp coconut flour
2 tbsp pumpkin puree
1 tsp pumpkin pie spice
Directions:
Mix together pumpkin puree in a large bowl, and almond butter until well combined.
Add liquid stevia, pumpkin pie spice, and coconut flour and mix well.
Make small balls from mixture and place onto a baking tray.
Place in the freezer for 1 hour.
Serve and enjoy.
Nutrition: Calories: 96 Fat: 8 g Carbs: 4 g Sugar: 1 g Protein: 2 g Cholesterol: 0 mg

503. Smooth Peanut Butter Cream

Preparation Time: 10 minutes
Cooking Time: 0 minutes
Servings: 8
Ingredients:
1/4 cup peanut butter
4 overripe bananas, chopped
1/3 cup cocoa powder
1/4 tsp vanilla extract
1/8 tsp salt
Directions:
In the blender add all the listed ingredients and blend until smooth.

Serve immediately and enjoy.
Nutrition: Calories: 101 Fat: 5 g Carbs: 14 g Sugar: 7 g Protein: 3 g Cholesterol: 0 mg

504.   Pumpkin Pie Trail Mix
Preparation Time: 5 minutes
Cooking Time: 0 minutes
Servings: 1
Ingredients:
½ tablespoon of pumpkin seed kernels
½ tablespoon of slivered almonds
¼ teaspoon pumpkin pie spice
½ tablespoon of Walden Maple Walnut or Pancake Syrup
1 sachet of Optavia Olive Oil & Sea Salt Popcorn
Directions:
Mix the syrup with pumpkin pie spice.
Get a quart-sized small bowl or resealable plastic bag to combine the pumpkin seed kernels, silvered almonds, Olive Oil & Sea Salt Popcorn. Trickle with syrup mixture.
Mix gently or toss together to make the popcorn evenly coat.
Per Serving: 3 Condiments , 1 Optional Snack

505.   Delicious Zucchini Quiche
Preparation Time: 15 minutes
Cooking Time: 60 minutes
Servings: 8
Ingredients
6 eggs
2 medium zucchini, shredded
1/2 tsp. dried basil
2 garlic cloves, minced
1 tbsp dry onion, minced
2 tbsp parmesan cheese, grated
2 tbsp fresh parsley, chopped
1/2 cup olive oil
1 cup cheddar cheese, shredded
1/4 cup coconut flour
3/4 cup almond flour
1/2 tsp. salt
Directions:
Preheat the oven to 350 F.
Grease 9-inch pie dish and set aside.
Squeeze out excess liquid from zucchini.
Add all ingredients into the large bowl and mix until well combined.
Pour into the prepared pie dish.

Bake in preheated oven for 45-60 minutes or until set.
Remove from the oven and let it cool completely. Slice and serve.
Nutrition: Calories: 288 Cal, Fat: 26.3 g, Carbohydrates: 5 g, Sugar: 1.6 g,Protein: 11 g, Cholesterol: 139 mg

506.   Cobb Salad with Blue Cheese Dressing
Preparation Time: 15 minutes
Cooking Time: 30 minutes
Servings: 6
Ingredients:
Dressing:
1/2 cup buttermilk
1 cup mayonnaise
2 tbsp Worcestershire sauce
1/2 cup sour cream
1 1/2 cup crumbled blue cheese
Salt and black pepper to taste
2 tbsp chopped chives
Salad:
6 eggs
2 chicken breasts, boneless and skinless
5 strips bacon
1 iceberg lettuce, cut into chunks
1 romaine lettuce, chopped
1 bibb lettuce, cored and leaves removed
2 avocado, pitted and diced
2 large tomatoes, chopped
1/2 cup crumbled blue cheese
2 scallions, chopped
Directions:
In a bowl, whisk the buttermilk, mayonnaise, Worcestershire sauce, and sour cream.
Stir in the blue cheese, salt, black pepper, and chives.
Place in the refrigerator to chill until ready to use.
Bring the eggs to boil in salted water over medium heat for 10 minutes.
Once ready, drain the eggs and transfer to the ice bath. Peel and chop the eggs. Set aside.
Preheat the grill pan over high heat. Season the chicken with salt and pepper.
Grill for 3 minutes on each side. Remove to a plate to cool for 3 minutes, and cut into bite-size chunks.
Fry the bacon in another pan set over medium heat until crispy, about 6 minutes. Remove, let cool for 2 minutes, and chop.

Arrange the lettuce leaves in a salad bowl and add the avocado, tomatoes, eggs, bacon, and chicken in single piles.

Sprinkle the blue cheese over the salad as well as the scallions and black pepper.

Drizzle the blue cheese dressing on the salad and serve with low carb bread.

Nutrition: Calories: 122 Cal, Fats: 14 g, Carbohydrates: 2 g, Protein: 23 g

507. Vanilla Bean Frappuccino

Preparation Time: 3 minutes
Cooking Time: 6 minutes
Servings: 4 servings
Ingredients:
3 cups unsweetened vanilla almond milk, chilled
2 tsp. swerve
1 1/2 cups heavy cream, cold
1 vanilla bean
1/4 tsp. xanthan gum
Unsweetened chocolate shavings to garnish
Directions:
Combine the almond milk, swerve, heavy cream, vanilla bean, and xanthan gum in the blender, and process on high speed for 1 minute until smooth. \
Pour into tall shake glasses, sprinkle with chocolate shavings, and serve immediately.

Nutrition: Calories: 193 Cal, Fats: 14 g, Carbohydrates: 6 g, Protein: 15 g

508. Dark Chocolate Mochaccino Ice Bombs

Preparation Time: 5 minutes
Cooking Time: 10 minutes
Servings: 4
Ingredients:
1/2 pound cream cheese
4 tbsp powdered sweetener
2 ounces strong coffee
2 tbsp cocoa powder, unsweetened
1 ounce cocoa butter, melted
2 1/2 ounces dark chocolate, melted
Directions:
Combine cream cheese, sweetener, coffee, and cocoa powder, in a food processor.
Roll 2 tbsp of the mixture and place on a lined tray.
Mix the melted cocoa butter and chocolate, and coat the bombs with it.

Freeze for 2 hours.
Nutrition: Calories: 127 Cal, Fats: 13g, Carbohydrates: 1.4 g, Protein: 1.9 g

509. Chocolate Bark With Almonds

Preparation Time: 5 minutes
Cooking Time: 10 minutes
Servings: 12
Ingredients:
1/2 cup toasted almonds, chopped
1/2 cup butter
10 drops stevia
1/4 tsp. salt
1/2 cup unsweetened coconut flakes
4 ounces dark chocolate
Directions:
Melt together the butter and chocolate, in the microwave, for 90 seconds.
Remove and stir in stevia.
Line a cookie sheet with waxed paper and spread the chocolate evenly.
Scatter the almonds on top, coconut flakes, and sprinkle with salt.
Refrigerate for one hour.
Nutrition: Calories: 161 Cal, Fats: 15.3 g, Carbohydrates: 1.9 g, Protein: 1.9 g

510. Optavia Fueling Mousse

Preparation Time: 3 minutes
Cooking Time: 3 minutes
Servings: 2
Ingredients:
1 packet Medifast or Optavia hot cocoa
1/2 cup sugar-free gelatin
1 tablespoon light cream cheese
2 tablespoons cold water
1/4 cup crushed ice
Directions:
Place all ingredients in a blender.
Pulse until smooth.
Pour into glass and place in the fridge to set.
Serve chilled.
Nutrition: Calories per serving: 156 Cal, Protein: 5.7 g, Carbs: 17.6 g, Fat: 3.7 g , Sugar: 4.5 g

511.   Tropical Greens Smoothie

Preparation Time: 5 Minutes
Cooking Time: 0 Minutes
Servings: 1
Ingredients:
One banana
1/2 large navel orange, peeled and segmented
1/2 cup frozen mango chunks
1 cup frozen spinach
One celery stalk, broken into pieces
One tablespoon cashew butter or almond butter
1/2 tablespoon spiraling
1/2 tablespoon ground flaxseed
1/2 cup unsweetened nondairy milk
Water, for thinning (optional)
Directions:
In a high-speed blender or food processor, combine the bananas, orange, mango, spinach, celery, cashew butter, spiraling (if using), flaxseed, and milk.
Blend until creamy, adding more milk or water to thin the smoothie if too thick. Serve immediately—it is best served fresh.
Nutrition:
Calories: 391
Fat: 12g
Protein: 13g
Carbohydrates: 68g
Fiber: 13g

Chapter 12:
28 Days Meal Plan

Day	Breakfast	Lunch	Dinner	Dessert
1	Eggroll in a bowl	Garlic Shrimp Zucchini Noodles	Avocado Lime Shrimp Salad	Tropical Greens Smoothie
2	Maple Lemon Tempeh Cubes	Shrimp with Garlic	Lentil Soup	Chocolate Bark With Almonds
3	Sabich Sandwich	Savory Cilantro Salmon	Mediterranean Bean Salad	Asparagus Green Scramble
4	Optavia Cloud Bread	Mini Mac in a Bowl	Butternut squash with Grapes	Healthy Broccoli Salad
5	Optavia Biscuit Pizza	Lean and Green Chicken Pesto Pasta	Mushrooms Stuffed with Tomato	Chicken Salad With Pineapple And Pecans
6	Broccoli Cheddar Breakfast Bake	Tomatillo and Green Chili Pork Stew	Chicken Cobb Salad	Cranberry Salad
7	Egg Stir Fry and Tomato	Chicken Stir Fry	Vegetables in air Fryer	Greek Yogurt Cookie Dough
8	Sabich Sandwich	Lean and Green Crunchy Chicken Tacos	Spicy Baked Tofu	Taco Salad
9	Herb Potatoes	Lean and Green Chicken Chili	Tomato Basil Salmon	No Bake Optavia Fueling Peanut Butter Brownies
10	Bacon Wings	Grilled Mahi Mahi with Jicama Slaw	Savory Cilantro Salmon	Chia Pudding
11	Cheddar & Chive Savory Smashed Potato Waffles	Tomatillo and Green Chili Pork Stew	Lean and Green Broccoli Taco	Pumpkin Balls
12	Peanut Butter Brownie Ice Cream Sandwiches	Mushroom Barley Soup	Lean and Green Garlic Chicken with Zoodles	Blueberry Muffins
13	Sabich Sandwich	Garlic Shrimp Zucchini Noodles	Lean and Green Cauliflower Salad	Delicious Brownie Bites
14	Eggroll in a bowl	Roasted Pork Tenderloin with Fresh Plum Sauce	Moules Marinieres	Pumpkin Pie Trail Mix
15	Broccoli Cheddar Breakfast Bake	Lean and Green Crockpot Chili	Cheeseburger Soup	Chocolate Bars

16	Optavia Biscuit Pizza	Mushroom Barley Soup	Vegetable Tofu Soup with Coconut Milk and Lemongrass	Cobb Salad with Blue Cheese Dressing
17	Optavia Cloud Bread	Garlic Shrimp Zucchini Noodles	Curry Roasted Cauliflower	Yogurt Berry Bagels with Cream Cheese
18	Egg Stir Fry and Tomato	Shrimp with Garlic	Sheet Pan Chicken Fajita Lettuce Wraps	Vanilla Bean Frappuccino
19	Sabich Sandwich	Savory Cilantro Salmon	Green Pea Guacamole	Tropical Greens Smoothie
20	Cheddar & Chive Savory Smashed Potato Waffles	Mini Mac in a Bowl	Lean and Green "Macaroni"	Chocolate Bark With Almonds
21	Bacon Wings	Lean and Green Chicken Pesto Pasta	Rosemary Cauliflower Rolls	Asparagus Green Scramble
22	Herb Potatoes	Tomatillo and Green Chili Pork Stew	Shrimp with Garlic	Healthy Broccoli Salad
23	Eggroll in a bowl	Chicken Stir Fry	Sheet Pan Chicken Fajita Lettuce Wraps	Greek Yogurt Cookie Dough
24	Optavia Biscuit Pizza	Lean and Green Crunchy Chicken Tacos	Alaskan Cod and Shrimp with Fresh Tomato	Taco Salad
25	Egg Stir Fry and Tomato	Lean and Green Chicken Chili	Salmon with Vegetables	No Bake Optavia Fueling Peanut Butter Brownies
26	Butter Brownie Ice Cream Sandwiches	Grilled Mahi Mahi with Jicama Slaw	Fresh Green Bean Salad	Chia Pudding
27	Maple Lemon Tempeh Cubes	Tomatillo and Green Chili Pork Stew	Mediterranean Bean Salad	Pumpkin Balls
28	Bacon Wings	Mushroom Barley Soup	Butternut squash with Grape	Blueberry Muffins

Conclusion

I know you're the type of woman who is constantly balancing things: work, kids, housework, hobbies. You take care of everyone else, but find yourself feeling drained and short on time to enjoy life too. At first, it seems like nothing ever changes or improves, even though you're working hard. But what if I told you that there was a way to eat delicious food that tastes better than anything you've ever eaten before AND save money? It's true; this cookbook was designed with YOU in mind! This book will show how to buy less expensive ingredients by shopping at your local farmer's markets or buying from wholesale clubs like Costco or Sam's Club. You'll be amazed by how much food you got for the money! You'll also learn how to prepare and store dishes that taste better than restaurant food, all while only throwing away what's leftovers. You'll feel proud of yourself when you look in the mirror knowing that your family is being nourished well while you save money.

I'm sure you're curious to know how much this book is going to cost you. You're not the kind of woman who believes in spending a lot of money on food, but that doesn't mean that you want to spend next to nothing. You want to get the most for your money while still eating delicious food. My goal was to make this book as affordable as possible so that you can read it and feel good about buying a healthier lifestyle for your family without breaking the bank. So, what do you say? Will you join me on my healthy cooking adventure this year? I'm sure you'll love it, and I'd love to hear all about your delicious discoveries as you save money.

In this Lean and Green cookbook, we talked about a ton of ways that you can save money on your grocery bill, as well as tricks to transform simple dishes into healthy miracles. All the recipes are easy, cheap, and quick to make. And you don't have to be a chef to make them!

Many of the recipes in this cookbook will give you the opportunity to eat tasty foods without any guilt. You will get all of the nutrients that your body needs on a daily basis, and it won't have all of those extra Calories: that you just don't need. Not having these extra Calories: will help you with your weight loss efforts or other weight-related goals, and this book can serve as one of your tools as you work toward them.

You will start to feel better as you learn how to include these foods in your diet, and you will enjoy how much better you look as a result of your healthier choices. You will find that surviving on a diet that is both lean and green can be much easier than you ever imagined. You can find all sorts of delicious recipes in this book that are designed to benefit you and your body in so many different ways. Many of the recipes in this cookbook are very healthy, but others are just for fun, which means there is something for everyone. To experiment with new ingredients, I cook a lot. Those who share my passion know that the kitchen is my favorite room of the house. Cooking makes me happy, it's relaxing and fun. If you don't feel like cooking alone, invite friends (or your significant other) to join you — it will be much more fun! No diet can survive without a healthy dose of variety in the dishes one eats.

You can easily do it as well! There is no need to eat the same thing every day, just go through your favorite cookbooks and choose a few new dishes to try out. You and your family will love these new recipes, and you can save time and money in the process.

Made in the USA
Monee, IL
17 March 2022